Acculturation, Obesity, Resilience in Black African

Ella O'Brien

Abstract

Obesity and obesity-related health problems are a growing concern for many immigrants in the United States. Immigrants may engage in unhealthy assimilation by adopting the health behavioral patterns of the host country resulting in negative health outcomes such as obesity. The problem that was addressed is that the relationships between acculturation, resiliency, obesity health risks and obesity have not been fully examined in the body of research utilizing the Reserve Capacity Model specifically for Black African immigrants living in the United States. The literature that examines the linkages between acculturation, resilience, obesity health risks, and obesity outcomes among Black African immigrants is sparse. The purpose of this quantitative correlational study using a survey research design was to ascertain whether the predictor variable of acculturation showed a significant association with two criterion variables, obesity health risk symptoms and obesity; and whether resilience acted as a moderator between acculturation, obesity health risk symptoms, and obesity among Black African immigrants living in the United States. The participants of the study were 55 Black African immigrants residing in Washington, DC-Baltimore, Maryland area; Boston, Massachusetts, or Chicago, Illinois. Results of the study indicated that higher levels of acculturation were associated with fewer obesity health risks. Higher levels of resilience were associated with the fewest obesity health risks when the participant also had high acculturation levels. Resilience moderated between acculturation and obesity health risk symptoms. Additional results showed that neither acculturation nor resilience significantly predicted obesity. Furthermore, resilience did not moderate between acculturation and obesity. Recommendations for future research include other cultural factors, such as the individual's native country, that may be associated with obesity and health problems

related to obesity.

Table of Contents

Chapter 1: Introduction

The topic of immigration has received significant legislative attention since 2011 (Appleby, 2012), and ongoing debates exist regarding healthcare access for those immigrating to the United States (US) (Berman, 2013). According to the Migration Policy Institute (2013), immigrants comprised 13% of the total US population in 2011. Most immigrants are in better health than their U.S.-born counterparts, and they tend to have longer life expectancies, fewer chronic and acute health problems, and a lower prevalence of injuries sustained by accidents than native bom Americans (Antecol & Bedard, 2005; Appleby, 2012; Venters & Gany, 2011). However, as part of the acculturation process, immigrants often adopt the health behavioral patterns of the host country that result in negative health outcomes, a phenomenon referred to as unhealthy assimilation by Antecol and Bedard (2005). A serious health issue for both native bom residents of the US and US immigrants is obesity (Singh, Siahpush, Hiatt, & Timsina, 2011). The obesity prevalence rate for American adults increased from 13.9% in 1991 to 27.4% in 2008 (Singh et al., 2011). In parallel, the obesity prevalence rate for immigrants in the US increased from 9.5% in 1991 to almost 21% in 2008 (Singh et al., 2011).

Since the mid-2000s, there has been substantial research on obesity among immigrants, the rationale being that acculturation and unhealthy assimilation is likely to influence obesity rates (Ade, Rohrer, & Rea, 2011; Buscemi, Beech, & Relyea, 2011; Choi, Hwang, & Yi, 2011; Delisle, 2010; Delisle, Vioque, & Gil, 2009; Goel et al., 2004). Indeed, a consistent finding in this body of research has been that length of time residing in the host country has been strongly associated with obesity (Choi et al., 2011; Kaplan et al., 2004; Yeh et al., 2009). Historically, Black African immigrants have been a much smaller population in America than Mexican and Asian immigrants (Delisle, 2010). However, as of 2011, there were over 1.1 million Black African immigrants in the US, and this population increased by 100% from the early 2000s to the early 2010s (Migration Policy, 2011). It is the fastest growing immigrant population in America (Migration Policy, 2011). Moreover, it has been posited that over 20% of Black African immigrants who currently reside in the US three or more years are obese (Ade et al., 2011; Migration Policy, 2011).

While acculturation factors have been linked to obesity in studies conducted with immigrants, only recently has the concept of resiliency been considered to play a protective role in lowering obesity levels within a theoretical acculturation and health framework specific to immigrants (Ade et al., 2011; Delisle et al., 2009; Goel et al., 2004). Borrowing from both acculturation (Berry, 1997) and the *Social Cognitive Theory* (SCT; Bandura, 2011), Gallo and Matthews' (2003) *Reserve Capacity Model* (RCM) posited that sociocultural factors of socioeconomic status and the cultural context, inclusive of acculturation, interact with personal resilience, as defined as one's psychological reserve capacity resources, to influence both health risks and health outcomes in immigrants. The increasing national focus on immigration and healthcare and immigration health, the substantial increase of Black African immigrants coming to the US, and the increasing rates of obesity occurring among Black African immigrants call attention to the need for studies examining the linkages between acculturation, resilience, obesity health risks, and obesity among Black African immigrants (Migration

Policy, 2011; National Obesity Observatory, 2011; Berman, 2013).

Background

Obesity has become a public health problem around the globe: worldwide obesity rates have doubled since 1990 to 1.4 billion in 2011, with obesity rates rivaling worldwide hunger rates (Baukol, Vierkant, & Levine, 2012; Flegal, Carroll, Kit, & Ogden, 2012; Stewart-Knox et al., 2012). The US has the highest worldwide obesity rate, with obesity affecting over 30% of the US population (CDC, 2012). Immigrant populations continue to grow in the US. As of 2011, immigrants comprised 13% of the total US population (Migration Policy Institute, 2012). Immigrants often engage in unhealthy assimilation by adopting the health behavioral patterns of the host country that result in negative health outcomes (Antecol & Bedard, 2005). Not surprisingly, one of the most common health problems in the 2010s for immigrants is obesity (Edberg, 2011). There are consequences of obesity on direct healthcare costs in the US to various programs such as Medicare, Medicaid, and Federally Qualified Health Clinics in that patients require more prescription drugs and more visits to hospitals and clinics (Pelone, Specchia, Venaziano, Capizzi, Bucci, Mancuso, Ricciard, & de Belvis, 2012; Portes, Light, & Femandez-Kelly, 2009). There are also negative consequences on health outcomes in that obesity has been known to reduce one's quality of life, promote the risk of certain diseases, and increase the risk of dying prematurely (Withrow & Alter, 2011). For immigrants, obesity becomes a problem when being in a new culture begins to adversely shape their dietary habits and level of physical activity (Ruesch & Volken, 2012). In terms of Black African immigrants who could become obese due to poor dietary habits (Renzaho, Swinbum, & Bums, 2008), this could place a burden on the healthcare system in that some immigrants lack resources and insurance and therefore become entitled to programs such as Medicare and Medicaid that cost taxpayer dollars (Portes et al., 2009).

Black African immigrants are one of the fastest growing immigrant populations in the US. As of 2011, there were over 1.1 million Black African immigrants in the US (Migration Policy, 2011). Despite an increasing presence in the US and an obesity rate of higher than 20%, Black African immigrants are considered to be an understudied population in health research in relation to other immigrant groups (Borch & Corra, 2010). The sparse literature that has examined obesity rates among Black African immigrants has found equivocal findings (Ade et al., 2011; Asgary et al., 2011). For example, researchers did not notice any significant relationships between immigration status and obesity in adult Black African immigrants residing in the US (Ade et al., 2011). In another study, researchers found that Black African immigrants who had arrived in the US came to the US being obese, which went undetected in their heritage country (Asgary et al., 2011).

Few studies have examined obesity rates among Black African immigrants utilizing the meaningful theoretical framework of acculturation, despite the numerous studies on the effects of acculturation on health risks in Black African immigrants (Freeman, 2002; Khawaja & Miller, 2012; Lum & Vandera, 2010; Renzaho et al., 2008; Souiden & Ladhari, 2011). Acculturation refers to the processes of cultural change that ensue when an individual interacts with others in another cultural environment (Berry, 1997; Dere et al., 2010). Researchers have often focused on the role of resilience in ameliorating the effects of acculturation for Black African immigrants

(Bledsoe & Sow, 2011; Obrist & Buchi, 2008; Sherwood & Liebling-Kalifani, 2012). However, only recently, via Gallo and Matthews' (2003) Reserve Capacity Model (RCM) have the constructs of acculturation, resiliency, obesity health risks, and obesity been examined within a theoretical acculturation and health framework specific to immigrants (Ade et al., 2011; Delisle et al., 2009; Goel et al., 2004). According to Gallo and Matthews' (2003) RCM, acculturation and resiliency are likely to play interacting roles to impact Black African immigrants' health risk and health outcomes, including obesity (Venters & Gany, 2011). Borrowing from the RCM model, the researcher determined if acculturation predicted obesity health risks and obesity, and if resilience acted as a moderator between acculturation, obesity health risks, and obesity among Black African immigrants living in the US.

Statement of the Problem

The problem that was addressed is that the relationships between acculturation, resiliency, obesity health risks, and obesity have not been fully examined in the body of research utilizing the Reserve Capacity Model (RCM: Gallo & Matthews, 2003) specifically for Black African immigrants living in the US. The RCM (Gallo & Matthews, 2003) has been examined with other immigrant groups such as with Hispanics, but not with Black African immigrants (Gallo, Penada, de los Monteros, & Arguelles, 2009; Howarter & Bennett, 2013). Black African immigrants are an appropriate group to study because historically, little research exists and they are one of the fastest growing immigrant groups in the US (Kamya, 1997; Ade, Rohrer, & Rea, 2011; Venters & Gany, 2011). Additionally, acculturation experiences have affected Black African immigrants' physical and mental health after they have resettled into a new country (Matheson,

Jorden, & Anisman, 2008; Renzaho, Swinbum, & Bums, 2008; Lum & Vanderaa, 2010).

Resilience has also become a means for Black African immigrants to cope with life

stressors. However, limited research exists on Black African immigrants and resiliency

(Matheson et al., 2008; Bartholomew, 2012; Sherwood & Liebling-Kalifani, 2012).

Finally, Black African immigrants must confront the emerging issue of obesity that

affects them upon arrival into the host country and after arrival (Renzaho et al., 2008;

Delisle, Vioque, & Gil, 2009; Asgary, Naderi, Swedish, Smith, Sckell, & Doorley, 2011).

It is for these reasons that a study on the variables of acculturation, resilience, obesity

health risks, and obesity for Black African immigrants is worthy of exploration.

Purpose of the Study

The purpose of this quantitative correlational survey research study was to

ascertain whether the predictor variable of acculturation was significantly predictive of

two criterion variables, obesity health risks and obesity and whether resilience acted as a

moderator between acculturation, obesity health risks, and obesity among Black African

immigrants living in the US. The sample for the study consisted of 55 Black African

immigrants residing in Baltimore/D.C metro area, Boston, Massachusetts, or Chicago,

Illinois. In consideration of one primary predictor variable, one moderating variable, and

eight covariates, and setting the effect size set at medium, $J7 = 0.15$, power set at 0.80, the

probability level set at < 0.05, the required sample size was 54 (Kelly & Maxwell, 2003).

A sample size of more than 55 participants was planned, but this sample size was large

enough to have the power to identify even minimal statistical effects (Kelly & Maxwell,

2003).

Theoretical Framework

In the proposed study, two primary theoretical frameworks were utilized: (a) Berry's (1997) Acculturation Theory; and (b) Gallo and Matthews' (2003) Reserve Capacity Model (RCM). In this section, both theories are discussed and pertinent research studies that have utilized these theories are discussed.

Berry's (1997) Acculturation Theory

Berry (1997) described that there are four acculturation stages that are neither linear nor progressive but depend upon the individual's desire to connect with the dominant culture. These stages are: separation, assimilation, marginalization, and integration (Berry, 1997). Separation takes place when individuals identify less with a dominant culture and simultaneously hold onto their heritage culture (Berry, 1997). Individuals stay attached to their heritage while simultaneously withdrawing from the dominant culture (Berry, 2010). Furthermore, individuals prefer to engage socially with members of the same ethnicity (Lerman, Maldenado, & Luna, 2009). There is an adverse relationship between the separation stage and the personality traits of being social and open-minded (Berry, 2010).

Assimilation takes place when individuals identify more with the ethnicity of the dominant culture and identify minimally with their ethnic characteristics (Berry, 1997). In this stage, individuals choose the dominant culture over the heritage culture (Berry, 2010). Individuals are completely immersed into the dominant culture but have minimized immersion into the heritage culture (Awad, 2010). An individual at this level might acquire the personality traits that consist of for example, being agreeable, friendly, and somewhat neurotic (Berry, 2010).

Marginalization takes place when individuals identify minimally with both the heritage and dominant cultures (Berry, 1997). Individuals at this stage do not wish to immerse in either culture (Berry, 2010). Therefore, they will neither guard former attachments to their heritage culture nor take on new attachments to the host culture. Consequently, there is a possibility that this group could feel isolated because neither group, the dominant nor the heritage cultures are accepting of them (Lerman et al., 2009). However, if the individual already feels discriminated from members of the dominant culture, it could be the very reason he or she originally chose to be in the marginalization stage to begin with (Berry, 2010). At the marginalization stage, one might possess certain personality characteristics, such as being impulsive, contentious, avoidant, and less emotionally intelligent (Berry, 2010).

Finally, integration takes place when individuals identify with the dominant culture and simultaneously hold onto their heritage (Berry, 1997). The degree to which ethnicity is similar to the host country's ethnicity will determine how well one reaches the integration stage (Schwartz et al., 2010). For example, if one speaks English before going to another English-speaking culture then integration will be easier (Schwartz et al., 2010). Those who seek to integrate will be better equipped to adapt psychologically (Berry & Sabatier, 2011). The personality traits and behaviors that assist an individual in reaching the integration stage are being social, open to new experiences, being able to accomplish tasks more easily, and having more emotional stability which lead to more success in an acculturation experience (Berry, 2010).

At the initial onset of acculturation theories, researchers believed that the objective in an acculturative experience was to reach the last stage of complete assimilation with only one trajectory to achieve this goal (Berry, 2010). Researchers assumed that individuals would ultimately assimilate and blend into the dominant culture (Gordon, 1964). However, this linear approach has proven to be too conventional, simplistic, and rudimentary to explain the multi-various levels within acculturation (Ryder, Adlen, & Paulhus, 2000). As a result, Berry (1974,1980) introduced a bidimensional model called the Acculturation Strategies Framework designed to account for the transition that takes place when more than one cultural background come in contact with each other on a routine basis (Berry, 1997).

There are two distinct dimensions to be considered in Berry's framework; the first being an individual's desire to maintain and to be identified with his or her cultural heritage, and the second one being an individual's desire to maintain contact and participation with the dominant culture (Berry, 1980,1984, 1997). Within these two dimensions, there are four stages: separation, assimilation, marginalization, and integration (Berry, 1997). Berry's model does have faults however, for example, one critic stated that Berry's Model was far too complex (Triandis, 1997). Other researchers have criticized Berry's method because there is a theoretical interdependency within measures which implies that high numbers on one measure will be followed by low numbers on the other three (Ryder et al., 2000). However, the multi-level relationships within all stages of acculturation can differ significantly, and therefore researchers can mistake the results and make incorrect assumptions (Ryder et al., 2000).

Gallo and Matthews' (2003) Reserve Capacity Model

The Reserve Capacity Model (RCM), developed by Gallo & Matthews (2003), is a health behavior model that utilizes concepts from Berry's Acculturation Theory (Berry,

1997) and the Social Cognitive Theory (SCT) (Bandura, 1977,1986, 2011) to address the

pathways that lead to health disparities among ethnic minority groups in the US. In the

RCM, acculturation is viewed as a sociocultural construct that influences health outcomes

in interaction with personal resilience factors, defined as *reserve capacity resources*

(Gallo & Matthews, 2003). The RCM is aligned with Bandura's (1977,1986,2011) SCT

premise that behavior is a function of the person interacting with his or her environment.

Within the RCM framework, resilience is an intrapersonal psychological construct that

can provide a buffer between the sociocultural context and the health risk behaviors and

health outcomes of the individual (Gallo & Matthews, 2003). The RCM is comprised of

three overarching components: (a) the sociocultural context, inclusive of both the

socioeconomic context and the cultural context, of which acculturation is a key indicator;

(b) personal resilience factors, defined as reserve capacity resources, and (c) health risks

and health outcomes (see Figure 1). Gallo & Matthews (2003) proposed that factors

within the sociocultural context are mediated or moderated by the reserve capacity

resources to influence health risks and outcomes in immigrant populations. In this study,

personal resilience (i.e., having reserve capacity resources) was considered as a

moderating variable.

Personal Resilience

Sociocultural Context   **Health Risk & Outcomes**

SES Context
-Individual
-Household

Cultural Context
-Ethnicity
-Nativity
-Generation
-Acculturation

Health Risks
Behavioral
-Physiological

Health Outcomes
-Morbidity
Disability

Figure 1. Rese™ Capacity Model (Gallo & Matthews, 2003).

Research Questions

For this study, acculturation, the predictor variable, was measured via the

Stephenson Multigroup Acculturation Scale (SMAS; Stephenson, 2000). Resilience, the

moderating variable, was assessed by the Conner-Davidson Resilience Scale (CD-RISC;

Connor & Davidson, 2003). In correspondence with the RCM (Gallo & Matthews,

2003), there were two criterion variables in this study: (a) obesity health risks and (b)

obesity. Obesity health risks were assessed by the Weight-Related Symptom Measure

(WRSM; Patrick, Bushnell, & Rothman, 2004). The measurement of obesity was a

composite scale of three indicators: (a) BMI, (b) waist circumference (in inches), and (c)

a single-item used in a national survey (i.e., National Health and Nutrition Examination

Survey [NHANES], 2012) inquiring about current perceived weight status. Participants

answered the obesity indicators question twice, the first time regarding the current time

period, and the second time regarding when they first immigrated to the US. The "past obesity" composite score was entered as a covariate in statistical analysis to remove any associated variance with the criterion variables of obesity risk and obesity: this allowed for a purer association between the predictor and criterion variables (Polit, 2010).

In accordance with the RCM (Gallo & Matthews, 2003), the variables of (a) socioeconomic status as the socioeconomic context indicator and (b) the cultural context variables of (a) participant native country, (b) participant native bom status, (c) immigrant generation status, and (d) the age and gender of study participants have been associated with obesity risk and obesity in studies with immigrants (Delisle, 2010; Fayombo, 2010; Stewart-Knox et al., 2012) and were controlled for in the statistical analyses (i.e., covariates). The following research questions and hypotheses were investigated:

Q1. To what extent, if any, does acculturation, as measured by the SMAS (Stephenson, 2000), predict obesity health risks, as measured by the WRSM (Patrick et al., 2004), in Black African immigrants who currently reside in the US, controlling for study covariates?

Q2. To what extent, if any, does resilience, as measured by the CD-RISC (Connor & Davidson, 2003), moderate between acculturation, as measured by the SMAS (Stephenson, 2000), and obesity health risks, as measured by the WRSM (Patrick et al., 2004), in Black African immigrants who currently reside in the US, controlling for study covariates?

Q3. To what extent, if any, does acculturation, as measured by the SMAS (Stephenson, 2000), predict obesity, as measured by a composite score (i.e., BMI, waist circumference, and perceived current weight status), in Black African immigrants who currently reside in the US, controlling for study covariates?

Q4. To what extent, if any, does resilience, as measured by the CD-RISC (Connor & Davidson, 2003), moderate between acculturation, as measured by the SMAS (Stephenson, 2000), and obesity, as measured by a composite score (i.e., BMI, waist circumference, and perceived current weight status), in Black African immigrants who currently reside in the US, controlling for study covariates?

Hypotheses

Based on the four research questions of this study, four sets of hypotheses are proposed:

H1₀ Acculturation, as measured by the SMAS (Stephenson, 2000) will not significantly predict obesity health risks, as measured by the WRSM (Patrick et al., 2004), in Black African immigrants who currently reside in the US, controlling for study covariates.

H1ₐ. Acculturation, as measured by the SMAS (Stephenson, 2000) will significantly predict obesity health risks, as measured by the WRSM (Patrick et al., 2004), in Black African immigrants who currently reside in the US, controlling for study covariates.

H2o. Resilience, as measured by the CD-RISC (Connor & Davidson, 2003), will not significantly moderate between acculturation, as measured by the SMAS (Stephenson, 2000), and obesity health risks, as measured by the WRSM (Patrick et al., 2004), in Black African immigrants who currently reside in the US, controlling for study covariates.

H2a Resilience, as measured by the CD-RISC (Connor & Davidson, 2003), will significantly moderate between acculturation, as measured by the SMAS (Stephenson,

2000), and obesity health risks, as measured by the WRSM (Patrick et al., 2004), in Black African immigrants who currently reside in the US, controlling for study covariates.

H3o- Acculturation, as measured by the SMAS (Stephenson, 2000) will not significantly predict obesity, as measured by a composite score (i.e., BMI, waist circumference, and perceived current weight status), in Black African immigrants who currently reside in the US, controlling for study covariates.

H3a. Acculturation, as measured by the SMAS (Stephenson, 2000) will significantly predict obesity, as measured by a composite score (i.e., BMI, waist circumference, and perceived current weight status), in Black African immigrants who currently reside in the US, controlling for study covariates.

H4o. Resilience, as measured by the CD-RISC (Connor & Davidson, 2003), will not significantly moderate between acculturation, as measured by the SMAS (Stephenson, 2000), and obesity, as measured by a composite score (i.e., BMI, waist circumference, and perceived current weight status), in Black African immigrants who currently reside in the US, controlling for study covariates.

H4a. Resilience, as measured by the CD-RISC (Connor & Davidson, 2003), will significantly moderate between acculturation, as measured by the SMAS (Stephenson, 2000), and obesity, as measured by a composite score (i.e., BMI, waist circumference, and perceived current weight status), in Black African immigrants who currently reside in the US, controlling for study covariates.

Nature of the Study

The proposed study utilized a quantitative correlational research design to examine the predictive relationship between acculturation, the predictor (independent) variable, and obesity health risks and obesity, the criterion (dependent) variables; and to determine whether resilience moderated the relationship between acculturation and obesity health risks and obesity. The predictor variable of acculturation was measured via the Stephenson Multigroup Acculturation Scale (SMAS; Stephenson, 2000). The moderating variable of resilience was measured by using the CD-RISC (Connor & Davidson, 2003). The criterion variable of obesity health risks was assessed by the 20-item Weight-Related Symptom Measure (WRSM: Patrick et al., 2004). The criterion variable of obesity status was assessed by three indicators, BMI, waist circumference (in inches), and self-reported perceived weight status, all of which have been validated and used as self-report indicators of obesity (Karasu, 2012; Lin et al., 2012; Rothman, 2008).

The sample for the study was a convenience sample of 55 Black African immigrants residing in Washington, DC-Baltimore, Maryland area; Boston, Massachusetts, or Chicago, Illinois. In consideration of one primary predictor variable, one moderating variable, and eight covariates, and setting the effect size set at medium, f^2 = 0.15, power set at 0.80, the probability level set at < 0.05, the required sample size is 54 (Kelly & Maxwell, 2003). A sample size of 55 participants was planned, as this sample size was large enough to have the power to identify even minimal statistical effects (Kelly & Maxwell, 2003).

The participants were recruited through the Africans' Universe foundation; a community-based foundation located in Boston, Massachusetts that provides outreach and services for African immigrants in Boston, Massachusetts and New York, New York; Research Chicago, an organization that recruits participants for studies; and Bethel World Outreach, a church located in Silver Springs, MD that has a very large congregation of

African immigrants. The researcher of this study established communication with the Africans' Universe foundation's director, established an agreement with Research Chicago, and established communication with the Executive Director of Bethel Church as the point of contacts who gave the surveys to study participants who met the study sample parameters inviting them to participate in the study. The researcher provided an email link to Africans' Universe and Research Chicago so that the Directors could send it to interested participants containing a consent form that the participant had to sign, as well as a link to the survey on SurveyMonkey™. Data collection was done via SurveyMonkey™. Participants through Africans' Universe and Research Chicago were sent a SurveyMonkey™ link via their personal email and they completed the survey by clicking on the link. The participants had two months to complete the survey.

Prior to conducting statistical analyses for hypothesis testing, descriptive information on the sample was computed. In addition, survey scales were computed and analyses were run for descriptive information on study variables. Specific statistical tests were conducted to determine and address any violations of assumptions for hierarchical multiple regression (Cohen, 1978; Polit, 2010). The study hypotheses was tested via hierarchical multiple regression analyses for moderation (Baron & Kenny, 1986; Frazier, Tix, & Barron, 2004).

In the proposed study, a quantitative correlational research design was optimal, as data was gathered from the study participants via self-report measures and statistical tests were conducted to capture the relationships among study phenomena (Kaplan, 2004; Vogt, 2007). A quantitative method was selected due to its preciseness in establishing statistical relationships among numerically-coded variables, allowing for a more objective assessment of the proposed model (Kaplan, 2004; Muijs, 2010). As data in this study were based on subjective responses of participants, neither a qualitative nor a mixed method research design was appropriate (Kaplan, 2004; Muijs, 2010). A survey research design was necessary as the personal factors measured in this study could not be manipulated by the researcher; in other words, the variables under examination in this study precluded the use of an experimental research design (Vogt, 2007).

Significance of the Study

This study is significant for practical as well as theoretical and research reasons. The data collected in this study helped to determine if resilience moderated between acculturation, obesity health risks, and obesity among Black African immigrants. Obesity is a serious health issue that affects over 21% of the immigrant population and over 20% of the Black African immigrant population in the US (CDC, 2012). An enhanced understanding of acculturation and the interactions between acculturation and resilience on obesity and obesity health risks for Black African immigrants can help to assist leaders of mental health and healthcare organizations that serve Black African immigrants to establish and provide educational and obesity prevention programs that address those factors of acculturation and resilience that play a role in obesity. For example, organizational leaders of immigrant organizations (as well as clinicians) will be able to create programs to reduce stress as it relates to acculturation and build resilience in Black African immigrants, which may prevent them from becoming obese and developing health problems resulting from obesity. Importantly, results from this study may help to promote health initiatives in Black African immigrant communities that can link individuals to needed healthcare services.

This study has numerous theoretical and research contributions. The study will contribute to acculturation and resilience theory by providing a better understanding of how acculturation and resiliency processes may influence health outcomes in a specific immigrant population, Black African immigrants. Perhaps the most significant contribution of this study is its examination of acculturation, resilience, obesity health risks, and obesity outcomes among Black African immigrants using Gallo and Matthew's (2003) RCM theoretical framework. To date, the RCM framework (Gallo & Matthews, 2003) has been tested only in Hispanic immigrant populations and on White women (Gallo, Matthews, Bogart, & Vranceanu, 2005). Finally, this study is important with regard to its contribution the minimal body of research that has assessed obesity rates in Black African immigrants (e.g., Ade et al., 2011; Asgary et al., 2011). While the study did not provide national rates of obesity among Black African immigrants, it did provide obesity health risks and obesity data on Black African immigrant samples in specific US communities.

Definition of Key Terms

Acculturation. Acculturation is defined as the processes of cultural change that ensue when an individual interacts with others in another cultural environment (Berry, 1997; Dere, Kirmayer, & Ryder, 2010).

Acculturation stress. Acculturative stress is a culmination of psychological and emotional agitation that ensues while one is attempting to acculturate because there is a need for adaptation to more than one culture (Albright, Harris, & LaFramboise, 2010).

Assimilation. Assimilation is a term used in Berry's Acculturation Theory that takes place when individuals identify more with the ethnicity of the dominant culture and identify minimally with their ethnic characteristics (Berry, 1997).

Body mass index (BMI). Body Mass Index is a way to measure body fat by calculating an individual's height and weight (Ward-Smith, 2010).

Integration. Integration is a term used in Berry's Acculturation Theory that takes place when individuals identify with a dominant culture and simultaneously hold onto their heritage culture (Berry, 1997).

Marginalization. Marginalization is a term used in Berry's Acculturation Theory that takes place when individuals identify minimally with both the ethnicity of the dominant culture and the ethnicity of the heritage culture (Berry, 1997).

Obesity. Obesity is defined as a Body Mass Index (BMI) of more than **30** or greater (National Institutes of Health, **2012).**

Obesity health risks. Obesity health risks are defined as poor health due to overweight or obesity as evidenced by symptoms such as fatigue, shortness of breath, back and joint pain, water retention, and frequent urination (Patrick et al., 2004).

Resilience. Resilience is defined as a protective factor in promoting positive adaptation to stressful life circumstances and it enables one to recover much more quickly (Greve & Leipold, 2009).

Separation. Separation is a term used in Berry's Acculturation Theory that takes place when individuals identify less with a dominant culture and simultaneously hold onto their heritage culture (Berry, 1997).

Unhealthy Assimilation. Unhealthy assimilation refers to the tendency for immigrants to converge or adopt unhealthy health behavioral patterns of the host country (Antencol & Bedard, 2005).

Summary

Immigration and healthcare reform have raised awareness of both the healthcare disparities among immigrants and the healthcare costs, including health insurance coverage, for immigrants (Appleby, 2012; Berman, 2013). Obesity is a significant healthcare problem that has become an epidemic in the American culture for both native bom and immigrant residents (Venters & Gany, 2011). Immigrants tend to become increasingly unhealthy as they acculturate to American society (Antecol & Bedard, 2005; Singh et al., 2011). The limited research on acculturation and obesity on Black African immigrants has lacked a cohesive theoretical framework and therefore the results of these studies tend to be ambiguous. For example, some researchers have found that Black African immigrants have higher rates of obesity than those who live in the host country, but on the other hand other researchers have found opposite findings (Gilbert & Khokhar; Ade et al., 2011). It is for these reasons that more studies are needed to add to the research base. According to the RCM (Gallo & Matthews, 2003), acculturation and resiliency are likely to play interacting roles to impact Black African immigrants' health risk and health outcomes, including obesity (Gilbert & Khokhar; Ade et al., 2011; Venters & Gany, 2011). This study will contribute to numerous bodies of literature (i.e., acculturation, resilience, obesity health risks, obesity) and is novel in its use of the RCM (Gallo & Matthews, 2003) via its testing of the theory in a sample of Black African immigrants.

The purpose of this quantitative correlational survey research study was to ascertain whether the predictor variable of acculturation is significantly predictive of two criterion variables, obesity health risks and obesity, and whether resilience acted as a moderator between acculturation, obesity health risks, and obesity among Black African immigrants living in the US. The researcher will provide a background on prior studies conducted on these topics, and will then describe the research method and design. The research method that was conducted was a quantitative correlational survey research design. The population of the study was 55 Black African immigrants who were either given a paper survey for completion, or sent a SurveyMonkey™ link via their personal email with a survey that they clicked on and completed. The researcher then collected the data via SurveyMonkey™ and conducted the analysis.

Chapter 2: Literature Review

The purpose of this quantitative correlational survey research study was to ascertain whether the predictor variable of acculturation was significantly predictive of two criterion variables, obesity health risks and obesity, and whether resilience acted as a moderator between acculturation, obesity health risks, and obesity among Black African immigrants living in the US. The literature review begins with a discussion on acculturation, with specific emphasis given to acculturation and health, and acculturation among Black African immigrants. A discussion of resilience follows, especially as it relates to Black African immigrants and their health. Obesity is the topic for the final section, with discussion devoted to obesity among Black African immigrants. A summary section completes the literature review.

Documentation

The researcher accessed key databases to retrieve relevant peer-reviewed scholarly works of research. The primary databases used were ProQuest Central, Academic Onefile, and Expanded Academic ASAP. The researcher found literature on various topics by typing in key words such as acculturation, obesity, immigrants, Black African immigrants, and resilience, and by combining topic words for a more precise search. In addition, the researcher used credible, governmental websites such as the Centers for Disease and Control Prevention (CDC) and the World Health Organization (WHO) for specific data and statistics related to the study.

Acculturation

Acculturation refers to the processes of cultural change that ensue when an individual interacts with others in another cultural environment (Berry, 1997; Dere et al., 2010). A multi-various procedure of transition occurs when more than one culturally different background come in contact with one another on a routine basis (Awad, 2010). From a psychological standpoint, acculturation is the consequence of cultural contact on a long-term basis in that the larger the cultural distance, the more the acculturative stress there will be (van der Vijver, 2008). The stages an immigrant will go through while moving from one culture to another consist of the following: (a) cultural shock, (b) irritating thoughts about the new culture, (c) reintegration into the new culture, (d) acceptance of the new culture, and (e) reciprocal interdependence in that the individual is able to live successfully amongst both cultures (Iliescu & Gheorghiu, 2011).

Acculturation and Health

When immigrants migrate to a new country, it can become stressful (Lum & Vanderaa, 2010). The link between acculturative experiences and health patterns is multifactorial (Helweg-Larsen & Standoff, 2008). Acculturation can have a significant effect on one's physical and mental health (Corral & Landrine, 2008; Zhang & Goodsen, 2011). The accumulation of stressful life situations can eventually take its toll on immigrants' health when they become elderly (Lum & Vanderaa, 2010). Disparities in ethnic and racial minority groups in the US have led to a diminished quality of life for some immigrants, in that they lack access to healthcare or prevention services and are subject to stress due to perceived discrimination by the host country (Eddy et al., 2010). This appears to be the case for Mexican-born immigrants in that they lacked healthcare resources (Carter-Pokras, 2008). Over one third of Mexican immigrants surveyed/studied, those under age 65 did not have health insurance (Carter-Pokras, 2008).

Acculturation plays a role in smoking, diet, cancer screening, physical activity, and morbidity; however the relationship between acculturation and health differ more strongly according to varying ethnicities (Corral and Landrine, 2008). For example, an increase in acculturation for Latino(a)s resulted in consumption of higher fat foods, although it was found to be the converse for African Americans (Corral & Landrine, 2008). An increase in acculturation for Mexican-born immigrants led to lower rates of obesity as compared to US-born Mexicans (Carter-Pokras et al., 2008). And Mexican-American immigrants had higher BMI scores and a greater tendency to become obese than their Asian American counterparts (Schaefer, Salazar, Bruhn, Saviano, Boushey, & Van Loan, 2009). Other factors associated with acculturation such as perceived discrimination and chronic discrimination have also led to increased abdominal obesity, according to an acculturation study on White immigrants of the Polish, Italian, Jewish, and Irish decent in the US (Hunt & Williams, 2009). Type 2 diabetes was more prevalent for Hispanic immigrants who were more acculturated and less prevalent for those who were less acculturated, however diabetes was not correlated to acculturation for Chinese immigrants (Kandola, Diez-Roux, Chan, Daviglus, Jackson, Ni, & Schreiner, 2008).

Helweg-Larsen and Standoff (2008) conducted an acculturation study on health

behaviors and determined that the more Bosnian immigrants adapted to the mainstream

culture, the more they understood the health risks of smoking. In another acculturation

study, religious participation for Mexican immigrants prevented the use of tobacco

products even as they became more acculturated and gained more education (Gillum,

2011). And in an acculturation study on smoking, Black African immigrants smoked less

than Black African Americans, but the authors noted the importance of early intervention

to prevent Black African immigrants from beginning to smoke (Bennett et al., 2008).

However, even though Black African immigrants do smoke less, those who do smoke are

at the same risk levels as Black African Americans in terms of severity of cigarette use

(Tran, Lee, & Burgess, 2010). Finally, Henken, Tucker, Gao, Falcon, Qawi, and Brugge

(2011) found that respiratory disease was strongly related to acculturation, depression,

higher levels of stress, and smoking for a sample of Puerto Ricans living in Boston, MA.

Acculturative Stress

When immigrants migrate to another country, the immigration process itself

might not be stressful, but the acculturation experience does prove stressful

(Bhattacharya, 2011). Acculturative stress is a culmination of psychological and

emotional agitation that ensues while one is attempting to acculturate because there is a

need for adaptation to more than one culture (Albright et al., 2010). It is burdensome on

an immigrant's capability to cope and generally creates anxious thoughts and feelings

(Chang, 2009). Acculturative stress develops because of language and communication

boundaries, incompatibilities between the heritage and dominant cultures, and feelings of

discrimination to name a few (Friedlander & Royt, 2008). It also creates feelings of inadequacy and desolation (Albright, et al., 2010). In the initial stages of being in a new culture, one can experience physical and psychological symptoms such as for example, losing sleep, feeling isolated, irritated, being distraught, and anxious (Iliescu-Gheorghiu, 2011). In one study, acculturative stress, smoking, and depression were significantly correlated to respiratory disease which indicates that acculturative stress can have an effect on one's physical health (Henkin et al., 2011). However, Bhattacharya (2011) conducted a qualitative acculturation study on immigrant men living in New York City who were originally from India and found that acculturative stress was mitigated when these individuals partook in social networking which led to social connectedness. In essence, social support played a pivotal role in lowering levels of depression amongst immigrant men (Bhattacharya, 2011). In fact, when Latino immigrant day laborers experienced acculturative stress, social connectedness buffered the adverse effects of acculturative stress on the overall health of immigrants (Salgado, Castaneda, Talavera, & Lindsay, 2012).

Disparities in ethnic and racial minority groups in the US have led to a diminished quality of life for some immigrants (Eddy, Isiordia, Jimenez, Martinez, McClure, McDades, & Snograss, 2010). The health of many immigrants tends to decline when they acculturate into the American society, and the amount of medical care that is accessible to immigrants plays an important role on the overall health of immigrants (Gorman, Ghazal Read, & Krueger, 2010). Researchers found that there was not as much access to healthcare or prevention services for immigrants, and there is an increased amount of stress because of perceived discrimination by the host country (Eddy et al., 2010).

The larger the cultural disparity, the more acculturative stress there will be among immigrants (van der Vijver, 2008). Depression is a dominant health problem for immigrants residing in the US and it is linked to acculturation (Choi, Miller, & Wilbur, 2009). Some of the factors found to cause depression for immigrants in addition to the acculturation experience are poor living conditions, unemployment, lower levels of education, and being separated from family members (Santiago-Rivera et al., 2011). In terms of depression, for a sample of Arab-Americans, as discrimination increased, depression increased, and therefore the degree to which Arab-Americans were unable to acculturate also increased (Aprahamian, Kaplan, Sutter, Visser, & Windham, 2011). In addition, depression or other psychosocial adjustment issues were mitigated when Chinese international students in the US remained more socially connected with other Americans (Zhang & Goodsen, 2011). This type of psychological adjustment seems true also in Native American Indians who, upon becoming psychologically adapted to both Native American Indian and White cultures, were far less likely to become hopeless and depressed (Albright et al., 2010). In a study of Korean immigrant women, those who were more marginalized had higher depression levels (Choi et al., 2009). This was attributed to findings indicating that immigrants who identify with neither the heritage culture nor the host culture tend to have a higher risk of mental health problems (Choi et al., 2009). When an immigrant utilizes self-control, he or she can prevent negative thoughts that affect his or her self-esteem and therefore eliminate the psychological stress that exists from discrimination while acculturating (Awad, 2010). However, this has not been successful for some Native American Indian adolescents because the culmination of acculturative stress has led to severe mental health issues such as, anti-social behaviors, low self-esteem, anxiety depression, and suicide (Albright et al., 2010).

Perceived Discrimination

Discrimination takes place when a person or people from a group are looked upon critically from others (Hadley & Patil, 2009). This could be for example, being a victim of prejudice, experiencing racist attacks or being insulted for being different (Veling, Hoek, Mackenbach, 2008). The brunt of discrimination, either perceived or real can have an immense effect on the overall health of those who are targeted by the discrimination (Lin, Li, Wang, Hong, Fang, Qin, and Stanton, 2011). Researchers found that discrimination may have an especially negative effect on an immigrant's mental health (Chae, Lee, Lincoln, & Ihara, 2012). For example, daily discrimination had a strong effect on the mental health of Asian immigrant men in the US, and this was especially true when they did not speak English very well (Leu, Walton, & Takeuchi, 2011). In another study, there was a positive correlation between perceived discrimination, and an increase in depression and cigarette smoking for Hispanic immigrant youth residing in Southern California (Lorenzo-Bianco, Unger, Ritt-Olsen, Soto, Baezconde-Garbanati, 2011). In another study, Veling et al (2008) found that perceived discrimination was positively related to lowering self-esteem for a sample of non-Western immigrants in the Netherlands. Perceived discrimination also had an effect on immigrants' physical health, for example, researchers conducted an acculturation study on White immigrants in the US, and found that as perceived discrimination increased, so too did obesity (Hunt & Williams, 2009).

The authors Lin et al (2011) conducted an acculturation study on the cross-sectional data of immigrants residing in China from the years 2004 to 2005. They found that discrimination was positively related to males who had more than one marriage, degenerative health conditions, shorter length of residence in the dominant country, and middle range of socioeconomic status. The authors also stressed the need for the reduction of discrimination against immigrants so that they could improve their over-all well-being and be a positive influence to society (Lin et al., 2011).

Berry (2010) determined that the degree to which individuals are discriminated against will determine whether they are eligible to participate in the larger society. Various factors predict the degree to which individuals will suffer from discrimination such as; language fluency, country of birth, monetary status, and religious affiliation (Hadley & Patel, 2009). When ethnic minorities interact with members of the dominant culture and they are stereotyped, they feel discriminated against because they are culturally different from the dominant culture (Albright, Harris & LaFromboise, 2010). For instance, individuals of Arabic descent and individuals of Middle Eastern decent in the US have experienced discriminating acts against them since the 1900's, however since 9/11 these acts have worsened (Awad, 2010).

Aprahamian, Kaplan, Sutter, Visser, and Windham (2011), noted that as discrimination increases, depression increases, and therefore the degree to which one has the ability to acculturate decreases. In another Arab-American ethnic study, Awad (2010) determined that individuals of Arabic and Middle Eastern descent living in the US who were of the Muslim faith were more discriminated against over those of the Christian faith, and religion was a high predictor of discrimination. Furthermore, since more Christian enclaves exist over Muslim enclaves, the American culture does not always recognize Muslim holidays in the same way as Christian ones, and therefore, despite Muslim Arab Americans' attempt to acculturate successfully, they are still being discriminated against (Awad, 2010). Individuals of the Jewish ethnicity from the former Soviet Republic honored their ethnicity when they used language as a buffer against discrimination by continuing to speak Russian amongst one another despite the chance that mainstream America could discriminate against them (Friedlander & Royt, 2008).

When ethnic minorities face more discrimination, they generally will hold even more strongly to their heritage culture, making them separate from the mainstream of the home culture, thereby using ethnicity to react against discrimination (Schwartz et al., 2010). In fact, feelings of perceived discrimination will push those of the same ethnic grouping more closely together to promote emotional wellness, confidence, and to feel more connected with others (Awad, 2010). In essence, when one identifies with his or her ethnic background, he or she is utilizing a protective strategy to offset the negative side effects that come from discrimination (Awad, 2010). Additionally, when immigrants formed social networks within their ethnicity amongst family and friends, mutual concern for each other was established which lowered levels of acculturative stress (Bhattacharya, 2011). Furthermore, family support proved to be a buffer against discrimination for a sample of immigrant Asians in the US and also mitigated depression (Chae et al., 2012).

Acculturation and Families

While some acculturation studies have emphasized variables such as gender, length of time in the new culture, and perceived discrimination, few studies have emphasized the importance of family in acculturation (Friedlander & Royt, 2008). Immigrant families endure many challenges when they resettle into a new country particularly with parenting (Renzaho & Vignjevic, 2011). Some parents send their children back to the home country if children become unruly while in the new country, believing that their children might not be strong enough to face the challenges of acculturation, and therefore sending them back will prepare them for the second arrival in the new country (Bledsoe & Sow, 2011). Other parents develop more strict controls, monitor children's activities more closely, and maintain a more authoritarian parenting style, thereby preventing a child from becoming too autonomous in an effort to protect them (Renzaho, Green, Mellor, & Swinbum, 2011). In some immigrant cultures, such as the Jewish community from the former Soviet Union, parents have tried to protect their children from discrimination of the host culture, and anxiety from being in a new culture which has resulted in a stronger parent-child emotional bond (Friedlander & Royt, 2008). Many families find that they must endure internal conflicts amongst individuals within the family when going through an acculturation experience (Leu et al., 2011; Moon, 2008). In one study, the researcher Moon (2008) analyzed family conflicts that arise between parents and adolescents during acculturation experiences. The sample consisted of over 300 Korean American adolescents. The results revealed that social support networks were essential in ameliorating strained relationships between parents and adolescents (Moon, 2008). In another study on family conflict, researchers found that for immigrant Asian woman, the relationship between family strife and mental issues was stronger when they had a strong sense of ethnic identity and concluded that the more central to an individual's own identity, the more likely an individual could experience depressive symptoms and anxious thoughts. This is because immigrant Asian women tend to spend longer periods of time at home with family members, and therefore do not interact as much with the outside world as Asian men by working outside of the home (Leu et al., 2011).

Acculturation and Risk Behaviors

The ethnicity of a group will determine whether it is a moderator of risk or resilient behaviors, particularly for Latino adolescents and substance abuse (Cox, Roblyer, Merten, Shreffler, & Schwerdtfeder, 2013). For example, when Hispanic adolescents were more aware of their own Hispanic ethnicity, it served as a protective measure against smoking and using substances, but had no effect on alcohol use (Unger, Ritt-Olson, Soto, Baezconde-Garbanati, 2009). However, in another acculturation study, researchers found that when immigrant Mexican adolescents were more sensation seeking and were more acculturated in the mainstream society of America, they were more likely to experiment with smoking cigarettes (Wilkinson, Okeke, Springer, Stigler, Gabriel, Bondy, Prokhorov, & Spitz, 2012). In terms of family intervention, Cox et al (2013) conducted an acculturation study on adolescent alcohol use and parental intervention and found that the more fathers were involved with their children, the less likely their children would use alcohol and the more acculturated they would be. However, mother involvement had no effect on the likelihood that adolescents would use alcohol and it did not affect the acculturation gap. In addition, researchers found that when Hispanic immigrant families lacked cohesion, Hispanic adolescents had higher risks of partaking in substance use (Unger et al., 2009). Taken one step further, when Hispanic adolescents spoke their native language in the home as opposed to English while acculturating in the US, families were less tolerant of delinquent behaviors (Saint-Jean, Martinez, & Crandall, 2008). Higher levels of acculturation may have a negative impact on the degree to which immigrants will partake in risk behaviors such as drug use (Akins, Mosher, Smith, & Gauthier, 2008). For example, Akins et al (2008) found that Hispanics who were more acculturated into mainstream society were 13 times more likely to use illicit drugs than their non-acculturated Hispanic counterparts. But according to an acculturation study conducted in the state of Florida, the authors found that although higher levels of acculturation predicted more substance use for Hispanic youth, this was mitigated through family support and intervention (Saint-Jean et al., 2008). According to Kulis, Marsiglia, and Nieri (2009), perceived discrimination was positively associated with substance use for a sample of Mexican youths in the US. In this regard, risk behaviors such as substance abuse were not attributed to higher levels of acculturation, but to acculturation stress brought about by perceived discrimination (Kulis etal., 2009).

Black African Immigrants and Acculturation

Historically, there has been little research on African immigrants in general (Kamya, 1997), and even less is known about Black African immigrants in the US (Borch & Corra, 2010). Black African immigrants remain a relatively understudied group in relation to other American immigrant groups (Borch & Corra, 2010). However, additional historical acculturation studies exist, focusing on Black African immigrants and African immigrants (Freeman, 2002; Kamya, 1997; Renzaho et al., 2008). For example, in one acculturation study on Black African immigrant children in Australia, the authors found that when children identified with their heritage culture and maintained healthy dietary patterns, they became more protected from obesity and chronic illnesses (Renzaho et al., 2008). In the US, an acculturation health study indicated that elderly

Black African immigrants reported poorer health conditions and higher levels of depression than elderly White immigrants; however the authors did not indicate the reason for this disparity (Lum & Vanderaa, 2010). One way that Black African immigrants protected their health more so than Black African Americans in the US was by smoking less than their American bom counterparts (Bennet et al., 2008). Even though Black African immigrants smoked less, for those who did were still at a similar risk as Black African Americans for severity of smoking (Tran et al., 2010). There was a significant correlation between acculturation, perceived discrimination, and substance abuse in Black African immigrants (Tran et al., 2010).

In one acculturation study, the authors examined the segregation patterns of Black African immigrants in the US and determined that Black African immigrants were more segregated from Whites, but only minimally segregated from native bom Blacks in the host culture (Freeman, 2002). One author examined spiritual well-being in relation to acculturation in African immigrants, (some of which were Black African immigrants in the US) and determined that spiritual well-being had a positive correlation with resilience as a coping mechanism for dealing with acculturative stress in the host culture (Kamya, 1997). Time related variables of acculturation such as length of time in the United States, and proportion of time spent in the US were significant for Black African Somali immigrant women who were carrying and delivering infants to full term between 1993 and 2006 (Flynn et al., 2011).

For some Black African immigrants, acculturation experiences were necessary as they had no choice but to immigrate to a new culture as a result of war and trauma in their heritage countries (Matheson, Jorden, & Anisman, 2008). Many Blacks in Africa have suffered from the injustices of decolonization and civil war (Bartholomew, 2012). Somali immigrants, after leaving their war-torn nation, experienced a great deal of acculturative stress upon arrival into Canada, and therefore had higher levels of stress hormones which made it more difficult to cope with the challenges of acculturation (Matheson et al., 2008). Some of the challenges they faced have consisted of stress that comes from acculturation, resettling into the new country, and discrimination from host country individuals (Ellis, Lincoln, MacDonald, & Cabral, 2008). In an effort to ameliorate some of these issues for immigrants coming into a new country, researchers conducted a study on 30 Black Somali and Somali Bantu adolescents who were newly resettled into America to see if they could benefit from a 4-tier mental health intervention program called Project SHIFA, or Supporting the Health of Immigrant Families and Adolescents (Ellis, Miller, Abdi, Barrett, & Blood, 2013). After 12 months, the authors determined that as a result of the intervention program, Somali and Somali Bantu adolescents' mental illness symptoms improved dramatically (Ellis et al., 2013).

South Sudan is also a country that has been plagued with civil war, taking the lives of approximately 2 million individuals over the last 10 years (Khawaja & Milner, 2012). It is for this reason that many of them have fled to other parts of the world such as Australia or neighboring countries to Sudan such as Egypt (Yeoh & Furler, 2011). Considering that an acculturation experience can have a negative impact on one's psychological state, it can also lead to strained family relationships (Berry, 2008). Khawaja and Milner (2012) conducted an acculturation study in conjunction with marital relationships of South Sudanese immigrant couples who had resettled into Australia. They determined that acculturative stress and lack of family support contributed to marital conflict as did tension—when South Sudanese women realized the freedom that Australian women enjoyed in a more egalitarian environment (Khawaja & Milner, 2012).

In another study on the impact of acculturation, researchers analyzed family relationships on a sample of African immigrants from Sudan, Somalia, and Ethiopia who had recently resettled in Melbourne, Australia (Renzaho et al., 2011). It is important to note that family disintegration within families during acculturation experiences are due to namely conflict between generations and roles (Hebbani, Obijiofor, & Bristed, 2010). African immigrant parents practiced restrictive parenting skills on their children which included instilling strict boundaries and maintaining close control which resulted in discouraged autonomy in their children (Renzaho et al., 2011). The implications of this research indicated that welfare programs in host countries must accommodate the difference in cultural parenting in an effort to help them develop their lives in the new culture (Renzaho et al., 2011).

As mentioned earlier on, Berry's four modes of acculturation are classified as the following: separation, assimilation, marginalization, and integration (Berry, 1997). Researchers conducted an acculturation study to understand the modes of acculturation in conjunction with consumer behaviors, which fall under the socialization category of acculturation, for West African immigrants in Canada (Souiden & Ladhari, 2011). The results indicated that West Africans fell into either the separation mode or the integration mode (Souiden & Ladhari, 2011). The separation mode takes place when individuals identify less with a dominant culture and simultaneously hold onto their heritage culture, and the integration mode takes place when individuals identify with a dominant culture and simultaneously hold onto their heritage culture (Berry, 1997). The implications of the study conducted by Souiden and Ladhari (2011) indicated that marketers must be aware that immigrant groups differ on consuming behaviors and that the degree to which immigrants' acculturate might not lead to a secure marketing strategy.

Resilience

Over the years, researchers have examined resilience by conducting studies from a variety of standpoints: psychological, sociological, psychiatric, biological, or genetic (Herrman, Stewart, Diaz-Granados, Berger, Jackson, & Yuen, 2011). They have recognized that studies on resilience are increasing rapidly (Herrman et al., 2011). Resilience is a relevant character strength that takes place when one uses protective factors such as positive emotions to adapt to negative circumstances (Greve & Leipold, 2009). When individuals have the character strength of resilience, they are determined to find purpose in life, and have the belief that they are capable of influencing their surroundings to reach more favorable solutions and grow throughout any experience in life (Bonanno, 2008). Resilience enables an individual to recover quicker after trauma or an emotionally trying event, which may result in growth under significant circumstances (Greve & Leipold, 2009). When an individual possesses resilience, he or she is capable of remaining stable during a crisis and has the potential to recover from it more quickly (Canetti-Nisim et al., 2009).

When an individual exhibits a more favorable approach to addressing problems in life, he or she tends to broaden his or her thought process and the result is the creation of resilience (Hart, Vella, & Mohr, 2008). Happiness is predicted by affirmative feelings, life satisfaction, and how well one copes with life situations, and finally, ego resilience is increased as daily affirmative feelings improve life satisfaction (Brown, Cohn, Conway,

Fredrickson, & Mikels, 2009). In one resilience study, the presence of resilience, ability and failure to remain resistant, and long-lasting stress were assessed in a sample of Arabic and Jewish immigrants (Canetti-Nism et al., 2009). The authors concluded that the best predictors of resilience and resistance were ethnicity status, minimal loss of psychosocial resources, greater economic status and social support, and minimal posttraumatic growth (Canetti-Nism et al., 2009).

In terms of mental health issues such as depression, when mothers were depressed and lacked psychological control, their children became more resilient (Malvar Pargas, Brennan, Hammen, & Le Brocque, 2010). In addition, a child's high intelligence quotient (IQ) proved to be a self-protective measure if they were born to a depressed mother (Malvar Pargas et al., 2010). Female breast cancer survivors who suffered from past trauma and psychiatric disorders experienced lower levels of anxiety if they possessed higher levels of resilience (Scali et al., 2012). And finally, among those who lived with and cared for family members with mental illness, factors that were used to promote resilience consisted of spirituality, religion, and other personal factors such as having loving, patient, and tolerant temperaments (Jonker, & Greeff, 2009).

The source of resilience comes from a variety of factors such as personality, positive thinking, hopeful attitudes, being resourceful, having the ability to cope, and the ability to be adaptable (Herrman et al., 2011). The Big Five personality traits that consist of the following: (a) being open to new experiences; (b) conscientious; (c) extroverted; (d) agreeable; and, (e) neurotic, have been linked to positive health results following adverse circumstances (Korotkov, 2008). For example, one author examined resilience in conjunction with the Big Five personality traits and determined that while there were positive correlations among many of the traits, conscientiousness had the strongest influence on resilience, followed by agreeableness, openness to experience, and extraversion (Fayombo, 2010). In addition, there was a negative correlation between resilience and neuroticism (Fayombo, 2010). Young people between the ages of 19 and 22 who scored high on neuroticism had a tendency to seek more social support in an effort to cope with difficult life situations (Ghimbulut, Ratinu, & Opre, 2012).

Language, tradition, and culture—the sense of belonging to a group, is positively related to higher levels of resilience (Kirmayer et al., 2011). In addition, identifying with individuals of the same ethnicity creates a higher sense of self-esteem (Edberg et al., 2011). For example, when orphaned children of Western Kenya owned goats through a donation program, it gave the children the ability to earn income as a result of managing the maintenance of goats, which provided a positive self-image in the children, and increased their resilience (Winsor, & Skovdal, 2011). In another cultural study on Canadian Aboriginals, resilience began on the outside of individuals based on the interactions among people and within cultures and communities (Kirmayer et al., 2011).

Researchers have found that spiritual well-being, resilience, and self-esteem are positively related (Gallo & Matthews, 2003). In a study on Korean mothers and daughters immigrating to the US, researchers explored the link between resilience and other factors such as self-esteem, having an optimistic outlook on life, being religious, being interdependent upon one another, and having a high regard for advanced education (Lee, Brown, Mitchell, & Schiraldi, 2008). The results indicated that both sets of women who experienced psychological affliction from tragedies, such as war, developed resilience when all of the other factors mentioned were applied (Lee et al., 2008). In a qualitative study on Bosnian refugee women who resettled into the US over a five year period, spirituality, family support, and community support helped them to create resilience (Soussou, Craig, Ogren, & Schnak, 2008). And finally, researchers examined the effectiveness of a self-help tutorial on resilience in order to mitigate symptoms of depression for a sample of 56 participants in Thailand, since depression has grown exponentially there (Songprakun & McCann, 2012). They found that the use of the self-help manuals moderated depression for the participants and even promoted recovery (Songprakun & McCann, 2012).

Developing Resilience in Adolescents

Self-reliance, goal attainment, and positive relationships are essential in developing resilient individuals for the betterment of our societies (Beightol, Carter, Gass, Gray & Jervertson, 2009). It is important to note however, that mental health issues affect over 20% of adolescents around the globe, some of which have stemmed from posttraumatic stress disorder, depression, or various other mental conditions (Hjemdal, Vogel, Solem, Hagen, Stiles, 2011; Wu, Feder, Cohen, Kim, Calderon, Chamey, & Mathe, 2013). This is a concern as adolescents need to grow up to be well-adjusted adults in order to function in society (Wu et al., 2013). Therefore fostering resilience in adolescents early on is a relevant way to strengthen them psychologically (Lee, Cheung, & Kwong, 2012). Researchers conducted a study on Norwegian students and found that higher levels of resilience minimized psychological disorders (Hjemdal et al., 2011). Some psychologists have indicated that resilience will develop naturally in adolescents who have grown up in adverse living conditions because many of them have had to deal with adverse life circumstances (Bonanno, 2008). In this regard, resilience is considered to be a contributor to the positive development of adolescents because resilience is induced when problematic situations come about (Lee et al, 2012).

There are ways to nurture students' resilience in classroom settings (Lee et al., 2012). For example, researchers conducted a quasi-experimental study on depression, low self-esteem, and low concentration in students who had been bullied in the classroom (Beightol et al., 2009). They found that when parents, teachers, or other adults enforced students with positive support like self-reliance and problem-solving skills, students had increased resiliency (Beightol et al., 2009). And in another resilience study conducted in New South Wales Australia, researchers found that when schools adopted intervention programs in their curriculums, students' levels of resilience had increased, and their use of tobacco products, alcohol, and marijuana decreased (Hodder, Daly, Freund, Bowman, Hazell, & Wiggers, 2011). When students develop attachments to teachers in addition to attachments to parents, it fosters resilience (Lee et al., 2012). Other ways to promote resilience in adolescents consist of: (1) providing love and support at home and in school, (2) nurturing positive relationships, (3) providing parental support and attention, (4) avoiding repetitious exposure to traumatic events, (5) preventing early entry into adulthood, (6) enabling self-efficacy, and; (7) providing stress training (Wu et al., 2013). The end result is that adolescents become resilient adults who are optimistic, can utilize positive emotions, be generous, be securely attached, be able to take sound risks, and be able to develop strong social ties with others (Wu et al., 2013).

Genetic factors may also have an effect on how resilient an individual can become (Binder & Holsboer, 2012). These genetic factors have the ability to generate resilient reactions to traumatic and stressful events, and may predict if an individual will be susceptible to mental illness into adulthood (Wu et al., 2013). However, each individual's genetic factors combined with developmental experiences will produce different resilience outcomes (Cicchetti & Roqosch, 2012).

Another way to promote resilience is by utilizing humor (Cheung & Yue, 2012). For example, researchers conducted a resilience study on Chinese students in Hong Kong and found that acculturative stress hindered students' adjustment in the new cultural environment, however humor helped to mitigate stress and therefore promoted resilience (Cheung & Yue, 2012). This is because humor has a sustainable quality in that it relieves anxiety, depression, and negative emotions (Cann, Norman, Welboume, & Calhoun, 2008).

Resilience and Black African Immigrants

Indeed, resilience has been known to be a self-protective measure for immigrants in minority status (Edberg et al., 2011). However there is limited research on immigrants and resilience (Sherwood & Liebling-Kalifani, 2012). With what limited research exists, it is important to discuss the coping mechanisms that enable Black African immigrants to endure an acculturative experience. For instance, one coping mechanism that serves both a cultural identity and foundation for healing after traumatic events is religion (Betancourt & Khan, 2008). Researchers have found that Africans, in general, gain strength through strong spiritual beliefs, and their philosophy of life is expressed through prayer and praises (Finley & Alexander, 2009). For example, spiritual connectedness enabled South African adolescents living in an institution as a result of HIV to cope with their adversity, and it allowed them to feel hopeful about their situation (Mohangi, Ebersohn, & Eloff, 2011). In one study on Somali adolescent immigrants in the US, researchers found that these individuals utilized religious services more frequently as opposed to mental health counseling when dealing with acculturative stress upon arrival into the new country (Ellis, Lincoln, Chamey, Ford-Paz, Benson, & Strunin, 2010).

Many Black populations in Africa have suffered many injustices due to decolonization and war (Bartholomew, 2012). This has made them suffer from psychological trauma (Matheson et al., 2008). In a recent study, researchers explored resilience in African refugee women residing in the United Kingdom who were originally from Somalia and Zimbabwe, had been subjected to violence, and had been affected psychologically by the trauma (Sherwood & Liebling-Kalifani, 2012). The researchers determined that these refugee women needed more treatment and support so that they could rely on their own resilience and in turn heal and reconstruct their identities from tragic events such as these (Sherwood & Liebling-Kalifani, 2012). In another study on Black Africans, Ovambo Namibians who were liberated from South Africa utilized personal resilience as their strength in helping them to overcome the struggle that took place during the decolonization of Namibia (Bartholomew, 2012).

War and conflict around the globe drastically change the lives of children who, as a result of war, endure separation from their parents, homelessness, and disability (Betancourt & Khan, 2008). For example, many Sudanese adolescents fled from their country in the 1980's as a result of war and violence in Sudan and resettled into the US, often times alone as their parents had been killed (Geltman, Grant-Knight, Ellis, & Landgraf, 2008). One protective process that aids in ameliorating the negative effects of psychological war trauma is social support (Betancourt & Khan, 2008). Social support can be for example, a psychosocial intervention that focuses on reestablishing an individual's prior living atmosphere prior to experiencing traumatic experiences such as war and violence (Betancourt, 2008). Social support consists of three main facets: (a) providing assistance in carrying out tasks, (b) providing guidance in carrying out daily activities, and (c) providing emotional nurturing (Betancourt & Khan, 2008). When events such as warfare are shared collectively as with the case for some Somalis, social support is increased which in turn enhances resilience (Matheson et al., 2008). Other protective sources are close ties to family and culture which enable children to be resilient to psychological trauma as a result of war (Betancourt, Brennan, Rubin-Smith, Fitzmaurice, & Gillman, 2010).

Migrating to a new country causes a great deal of stress (Obrist & Buchi, 2008). Therefore, resettling into a new country has led to the development of mental health issues in addition to the psychological trauma immigrants have already experienced prior to arrival in the new country (Matheson et al., 2008; Ellis, Abdi, Barrett, Miller, & Blood, 2013). For example, Somali children, after resettlement, suffered from acculturation stressors such as discrimination and stress from resettling which led to mental health trauma (Ellis, Lincoln, MacDonald, & Cabral, 2008). It is for these reasons that researchers launched a multi-level resilience building model that would enable Somali children to recover from psychological duress (Ellis et al., 2013). Over a 12 month time frame, the researchers found that the model provided the resources and support that helped to ameliorate depression and trauma for Somali participants (Ellis et al., 2013).

In collegiate level institutions, second generation Black African immigrants developed resilience against discrimination by maintaining their cultural identity and remaining connected to the opportunity framework of the dominant culture (Owens & Lynch, 2012). The study revealed that resilience prevented Black African immigrants from becoming susceptible to discrimination (Owens & Lynch, 2012). In addition to discrimination, Black African immigrants have endured other adversities while in the new country that consist of for example, personal relation problems in that some immigrants faced unsuccessful marriages, lack of work, working too much, or working in jobs that were physically exhausting to provide for the family, poor living conditions, and lack of being socially recognized in that their professional backgrounds were not respected (Obrist & Buchi, 2008).

In one particular resilience study on Black African immigrants in Switzerland, these immigrants experienced more stress upon arrival in the new country. However, they were able to adjust by developing life skills that enabled them to master the stress with the use of resilient behaviors (Obrist & Buchi, 2008). West African immigrant parents believed that they were developing resilience in their children when they sent them back to Africa (Bledsoe & Sow, 2011). This is because they believed that children who become unruly in the new country might not be strong enough to face the challenges of acculturation and therefore, sending the children back to Africa prepares them for the second arrival in the new country (Bledsoe & Sow, 2011).

Obesity

Obesity has become an increasingly important public health problem both in the US and globally (Centers for Disease Control and Prevention [CDC], 2009; Stewart et al., 2012). Obesity has increased worldwide in both developing and developed countries (Lokuruka, 2013). Obesity is defined as an excessive fat accumulation that poses a risk to health, and a Body Mass Index equal to or greater than 30 (World Health Organization [WHO], 2012). According to the WHO (2012), worldwide obesity has more than doubled. The CDC (2012) indicated that as of 2009-2010, 35.9% of Americans 20 years and older were obese. Flegel et al (2012) conducted an obesity study using the National Health and Nutrition Examination Survey (NHANES) and determined that from 2009 to 2010, obesity was 35.5% among men, and 38.8% among women. This percentage has not changed from a previous study conducted for the period from 2003 to 2008.

Obesity rates have been attributed to harmful lifestyle practices (Stewart-Knox, et al., 2012). Among factors leading to obesity is lack of physical activity, poor dietary patterns, over consumption of foods high in fat and carbohydrates, and urbanization (Lokuruka, 2013). There are numerous health risks associated with obesity, such as type 2 diabetes, hypertension, heart disease, osteoarthritis, stroke, and sleep apnea (Afitab, Kumar, & Barber, 2013; McVeigh, Gibson, & Hamilton, 2013; Turanjanin, Jovicevic, Bozic, & Zarkov, 2012). In addition, there is an increased risk of colon, breast, endometrium, and esophagus cancers (Moreley, Wakefield, Dulop, & Hill, 2009). Urologic disorders such as renal diseases, and prostate, kidney, bladder, and testicular cancers have also been linked to obesity (Ward-Smith, 2010). Some psychological disorders linked to obesity are low self-esteem, depression, eating disorders, and distorted self-image (Bjomelv, Nordahl, & Holmen, 2011; Incledon, Wake, & Hay, 2011). In some cases, obesity can even cause premature death (Mehta, & Chang, 2009).

Obesity: A Global Epidemic

Considering that obesity has become a global health problem, many studies have been conducted on adults in various communities around the globe (Aballay, Eynard, del Pilar Diaz, Navarro, & Munoz, 2012; Manuel, Lesmes, Marset, Izquierdo, Sala, Salas-Salvado, 2012; Wang, Wang, Liu, Wang, Liu, Zhao, Huang, Liu, Sun, & Dong, 2012). For example, researchers conducted an obesity study on over 25 thousand urban Chinese adults in Northeast China and determined that obesity has become an epidemic; however the risk factors differed between genders (Wang et al., 2012). Men who had higher levels of education and higher incomes were more apt to become obese, however women who had higher levels of education and higher family incomes were less apt to become obese (Wang et al., 2012). And in another study, the researchers analyzed obesity, metabolic syndrome, and cardiovascular disease in several South American countries (Aballay et al., 2012). The authors found that obesity and cardiovascular disease were highly associated with advanced age and poor lifestyle choices, that obesity led to cancer in the Southern Cone of South America, and that metabolic syndrome was highest in Chili, but less in Equador and in other areas (Aballay et al., 2012). In another South American study, researchers found that sugar intake was positively associated with obesity and lifestyles of inactivity in a sample of Brazilian participants (Penatti, Lira, Katashima, Rosa, & Pimenal, 2012). A European study on Portuguese adults between the ages of 18 and 103 revealed that lower levels of education were positively associated with abdominal obesity, and that of the representative sample of over 9,000 individuals, two thirds of population were obese (Sardinha, Santos, Silva, Coelho-e-Silva, Raimundo, Moreira, Santos, Vale, Baptista, & Mota, 2012). Researchers also conducted an obesity study on women of the Tangkhul Naga tribe of Manipur, India and found that as the socioeconomic status of younger women improved, they were more apt to become obese, and it was the converse for younger women of lower socioeconomic status in that they did not become obese. The researchers noted that expanded urbanization led to a change in nutritional intake, less physical activity, and more of a predominance of obesity (Mungreiphy & Kapoor, 2010).

Obesity and Children

It is important to mention children and obesity since children who are obese have the potential for becoming obese adults (Phillips, 2012). Childhood obesity has become a worldwide public health problem over the last several decades (Branscum & Sharma, 2011; Raj, 2012). It has particularly increased with immigrant minority children (Sussner, Lindsay, Greaney, & Peterson, 2008). Obesity in childhood poses a significant risk for diseases that affect major organs that can eventually lead to morbidity and mortality (Lubans, Morgan, Dewar, Collins, Plotnikoff, Okely, Batterham, Finn, & Callister, 2010; Raj, 2012). Some of the diseases that could affect children into adulthood as a result of obesity consist of cardiovascular diseases, hypertension, metabolic issues, Type 2 diabetes, and sleep apnea to name a few (Raj, 2012).

The causes of obesity in children are varied and consist of home and school atmospheres, lack of physical education and inactivity, lack of access to larger grocery stores, and poor dietary habits (Branscum & Sharma, 2011). Some studies conclude that children who come from lower socioeconomic households and/or ethnic minority households have poorer dietary habits (Pearson, Biddle, & Gorely, 2009; Beech, Fitzgibbon, Resnicow, Whitt-Glover, 2011; Liu, Jones, Sun, Probst, Merchant &

Cavicchia, 2012). On the other hand, there have been many children who have lacked socioeconomic resources yet have managed to consume nutritious foods, in effect demonstrating a dietary resilience (Stephens et al., 2011).

Family atmosphere has a tremendous influence on how dietary patterns develop in youths (Pearson et al., 2009). Parents with obesity become a risk factor to their children to become obese in that they model negative parental behaviors (Svensson, Jacobsson, Fredriksson, Danielsson, Sobko, Schioth, & Marcus, 2011). And parents who do not recognize when their child is overweight exacerbate the problem of obesity in their children (Phillips, 2012). However, when parents provide better support networks, enforce rules to promote better eating behaviors, and demonstrate healthy eating behaviors, their children will choose more nutritious foods and therefore prevent unhealthy weight gain (Pearson et al., 2009). Researchers conducted a longitudinal study on children between the ages of 7 and 15 who had obese parents (Svensson et al., 2011). They found that obesity in parents had a stronger effect on children as they grew older, however the age of onset of obesity was of less importance (Svensson et al., 2011). It is for this reason that parents need to exhibit positive dietary behaviors so that their children will model their behavior (Pearson et al., 2009).

Intervention

Treating obesity is a great challenge (Svensson et al., 2011). However, neglecting to treat obesity in children could result in a dire public health situation in the years to come (Raj, 2012). Proper nutrition is important in preventing obesity (Stephens, McNaughton, Crawford, MacFarlane, & Ball, 2011). For example, researchers determined that when parents modeled proper nutritional intake, their children ate more fruits and vegetables and made healthier food choices (Pearson et al., 2009). Self-control could be a relevant factor in developing better behaviors to limit the intake of sugary snack foods (Branscum & Sharma, 2011). Some of the ways to change eating behaviors in children include parent involvement, interactive educational programs during school hours, physical activity, and changes in nutrition (Nixon, Moore, Douthwaite, Gibson, Vogele, Kreichauf, Wildgruber, Manios, & Summerbell, 2012). Intervention programs that included behavior changing strategies were effective in preventing immense weight gain for teen girls (Lubans et al., 2010). Some of the techniques that were effective included; sport sessions during school hours and at lunch time, nutrition education sessions, parental newsletters, and social support via text messages (Luban et al., 2010). Interventions must be culturally sensitive so that they target individuals from various ethnicities and races and at earlier ages in schools, such as with elementary students since the chances for becoming obese increase as children get older (Long et al., 2012).

Obesity in the United States

In addition to it being a widespread epidemic in adults and children around the globe, obesity is also an epidemic in the US affecting over two-thirds of the population (Flegal, Carroll, Kit, & Ogden, 2012; Baukol, Vierkant, & Levine, 2012). Obesity has increased significantly amongst various races however it has a disproportionate effect on individuals of certain races (Kirby, Lian, Chen, & Wang, 2012). For example, around 50% of African-American women suffer from obesity as opposed to around 33% of White American Women (Flegel et al., 2010). And Mexican and non-Hispanic African Americans may be more affected by obesity than non-Hispanic White Americans (Long, Mareno, Shabo, & Wilson, 2012). Researchers conducted a study on Native Americans and found that obesity affected approximately half of Native American children living on reservations and in urban settings and attributed it to lack of physical activity (Baukol et al., 2012).

In a community based study on individuals of various races and ethnicities living in the US, the authors found that communities with different race and ethnic compositions were at a higher risk for obesity, but that it varied by individuals' race and ethnicity (Kirby et al., 2012). For example, Hispanic and non-Hispanic White individuals living in Hispanic communities had higher chances of becoming obese than did Asians and non-Hispanic Whites living in Asian American communities (Kirby et al. 2012). Researchers conducted an African American study to compare the effect of sleep deprivation and obesity for African American adult women from the ages of 30-65 (Bidulescu, Din-Dzietham, Coverson, Chen, Meng, Buxbaum, Gibbons, & Welch, 2010). The authors concluded that sleep disturbances caused by stress were linked to obesity for African American women (Bidulescu et al., 2010).

Immigrants and Obesity

Immigrant populations continue to grow in developed countries (Delisle, Vioque, & Gil, 2009). In years to come, the population of the US will continue to become increasingly diverse (Edberg, Cleary, & Vyas, 2011). According to the Migration Policy Institute, immigrants consisted of 13% of the total US population as of 2011 (Migration Policy Institute, 2012). There are health disparities among various immigrant groups in that some have better health than others, but one of the most common health problems for all is obesity (Edberg et al., 2011). However, in the last few decades, obesity has increased significantly in immigrant ethnic minority groups (Choi, Hwang, & Yi, 2011).

For example, researchers examined a sample of Mexican-Americans and a sample of Asian-Americans and found that the Mexican group tended to have higher BMI's and more instances of being overweight than did its Asian counterpart (Schaefer et al., 2009). On the other hand, according to the National Health and Nutrition Examination Survey (NHANES) data from 2001-2006, among Mexican immigrants in the US, Mexican immigrant woman had lower rates of obesity over Spanish speaking American-born women, but higher rates of obesity over American-born English speaking women (Guendelman, Fernandez, Thornton, & Brindis, 2011).

Obesity has been found to contribute to serious health diseases and has been associated with the acculturative experiences of immigrants in particular (Buscemi, Beech, & Relyea, 2011). Upon arrival into the host country, many immigrants are significantly less likely to be overweight and obese than their nationally-born counterparts (Roshania, Venkat Narayan, & Oza-Frank, 2008). Taken one step further, immigrants are far less likely to be obese than American-bom individuals (Choi et al., 2011). In fact, initially, they have better heath overall as compared to those who were nationally-born (Singh-Setia, Quesnel-Valley, Abrahamowicz, Tousignant, & Lynch, 2009). However, this has been found to change as the length of residence in the host country increases (Oza-Frank, Stephenson, & Venkat Narayan, 2011). There is a health paradox in that immigrants, upon arrival, are healthier than individuals bom in the host country, but they tend to lose this advantage over time (Edberg et al., 2011). For example, the longer Mexican immigrants resided in the US, the more they engaged in non-healthy dietary patterns (Carter-Pokras et al., 2008). But length of residence was not positively associated with obesity for immigrants from Europe, the US, Canada, and

Latin America living in Madrid, Spain concluding that immigrants are not overly exposed to factors that encourage obesity in Spain (Gutierrez-Fisac, Marin-Guerrero, Regidor, Guallar-Castillo, Banegas, & Rodriguez-Artalejo, 2009). Among Hispanic women in general, obesity was related to length of residence in the host culture, but was not related to low language acculturation or the level at which an immigrant is familiar with the language of the host culture (Wolin, Colangelo, Chiu, & Gapsture, 2009). In Canada, researchers conducted a study to determine if the BMI of various immigrant groups increased and converged with that of native born Canadians over a 12-year time frame (Singh-Setia et al., 2009). The researchers found that not all immigrant groups experienced the same results. For example, men from Non-white immigrant groups had a lower BMI over Canadian-born men, but men from White immigrant groups had similar BMIs as their Canadian-born counterparts, concluding that there are disparities in BMI changes for immigrants of White or Non-white descent (Singh-Setia, et al., 2009).

In one study, Latina mothers of overweight families reported that the food choices in their native countries were much more conducive to healthier diets (Sussner et al., 2008). The same was true for Liberian immigrants who noted that they had better access to healthier food choices such as fruits and vegetables in their heritage country (Patil, Hadley, & Djona Nahayo, 2009). Researchers conducted a study on diet acculturation for Ethiopian immigrant women residing in Israel. The aim of the study was to examine dietary habit changes for immigrants who migrated to more developed countries. The results indicated that after residing in Israel for several years, Ethiopian women had an increase in body mass, and they consumed more foods high in sugar and fewer healthy foods such as fruits and vegetables, concluding that immigrants face a much higher risk for obesity related diseases as a result of migration to a developed country (Regev-Tobias, Reifen, Endevelt, Havkin, Cohen, Stem, & Stark, 2012). In addition, even immigrant children are affected and have a greater risk for becoming obese than non-immigrant children if they come from lower income families that cannot afford to purchase healthier foods such as fruits and vegetables (Buscemi et al., 2011). On the other hand, Singh, Kogan, and Yu (2009) conducted a study on immigrant children and obesity, and found that the odds of becoming obese were 26% lower for children of immigrants as opposed to children of non-immigrants. The patterns for obesity varied among ethnicities and generation in the country. Despite this, the prevalence of obesity tends to vary for individuals of first and second generational status (Hosper, Nicolaou, Valkengoed, Nierkens, & Stronks, 2011). Researchers have concluded that immigrant BMI increases in advanced generations (Bates et al., 2008). In addition, there appears to be a positive correlation between higher socioeconomic positions, i.e. higher levels of education, and immigrant obesity for women, but not for men in countries such as Morocco (Hosper et al., 2011).

The transition from the nutrition of the heritage culture to the nutrition of the host culture has proven to have adverse side effects leading to obesity, Type 2 diabetes, and cardiovascular disorders (Delisle, 2010). In fact, for immigrant groups in particular, obesity augments the risk of chronic diseases such as heart disease and high blood pressure (Ade, Rohrer, & Rea, 2011). The farther African immigrants moved away from traditional foods, the more likely they were to consume foods that would lead to obesity and become less physically active (Renzaho et al., 2008). Immigrants who come to the US may lack familiarity with American grocery stores and may therefore be uninformed about the health risks of foods high in calories and low in nutrients (Van Hook & Baker, 2010). In a study of age at arrival and obesity, immigrants who arrived in the host country 20 years old or younger and remained there for more than 15 years were 11 times more likely to be obese than immigrants 20 years old or younger who had lived in the US less than one year (Roshana et al., 2008). However, immigrants who had arrived in the host country at age 50 or older showed no difference in the prevalence of obesity (Roshana et al., 2008). Therefore, the authors concluded that immigrants 20 years of age or younger are at a higher risk for obesity than those who arrive in the host country at older ages (Roshana et al., 2008). In another study on immigrants, obesity rates were twice as high for Latina immigrant women living in the US for more than 20 years as opposed to those living in the US for less than 10 years (Wolen, Colangele, Chiu, & Gapstur, 2009).

Researchers examined generational status, socioeconomic status, and gender for Turkish and Moroccan individuals living in the Netherlands (Hosper et al., 2011). Results indicated that women of a second generational status were far less obese than their first generational status counterparts. This was attributed to higher socioeconomic status. This pattern was reversed in men, although it was also attributed to socioeconomic status (Hosper et al., 2011).

Living in certain neighborhoods could explain why there are ethnic differences in obesity (Nicholson & Browning, 2012). Researchers concluded that neighborhoods where the social atmosphere was more agreeable were positively associated with children's physical activity (Franzini, Elliott, Cuccaro, Schuster, Gilliland, Grunbaum, Franklin, & Tortolero, 2009). Neighborhoods may have an impact on the degree to which one becomes obese because certain neighborhoods provide more access to food markets where healthier food options are available, as opposed to other neighborhoods that have only fast food restaurant options (Grafova, Freedman, Kumar, & Rogowski, 2008). Individuals who owned a car and lived in neighborhoods with more fast food restaurants tended to have a higher BMI than those who did not for a sample of participants living in Los Angeles, California (Inagami, Cohen, Brown, & Asch, 2009).

When researchers conducted a study on dietary patterns and the effect of neighborhoods for Hispanic immigrant women living in New York City, they found that when immigrants lived in densely populated areas with fast food restaurants, they were less likely to adhere to a healthy diet (Park, Neckerman, Quinn, Weiss, Jacobson, & Rundle, 2010). On the other hand, eating healthier food choices was positively linked to Hispanic women living in linguistically isolated neighborhoods where Spanish was spoken (Park et al., 2010). Newly arrived immigrants in Canada of lower income backgrounds who lived in neighborhoods that were more walkable and had more fast food restaurants tended to develop obesity related diseases more so than native born Canadians (Booth, Creatore, Moineddin, Bozdyra, & Weyman, 2013). And living in economically disadvantageous neighborhoods increased the risk for obesity in adolescent ethnic females, but had no effect on adolescent ethnic males (Nicholson & Browning, 2012). For Latino neighborhoods in Utah, higher socioeconomic status was significantly related to lower instances of obesity however residential isolation, or living in remote places, was related to higher instances of obesity (Wen & Maloney, 2011). Street connectivity refers to the degree to which streets connect to each other, and the denseness of intersections (Mercredy, Pickett, & Janssen, 2011). For adults 55 years and older, men who lived in areas where there was a high concentration of immigrants tended to have more risk for obesity, and women were less likely to be obese where there was more street connectivity (Grafova et al., 2008). Researchers conducted a study on two different ethnic groups in deprived neighborhoods in Sweden (Faskunger, Eriksson, Sven-Erik Johansson, Sundquist, & Sundquist, 2009). The study revealed that Middle Eastern immigrant women had higher rates of obesity over Swedish women who lived in economically deprived neighborhoods, and had higher levels of economic difficulties, which stresses the need for obesity prevention intervention programs for immigrant populations (Faskunger et al., 2009).

Black African Immigrants and Obesity

It is important to examine obesity, or lack thereof, in Black African immigrants. Black African immigrants have proven to be one of the fastest growing immigrant groups in the US, and the numbers continue to increase each year (Venters & Gany, 2011). Previous studies have focused on Black African American non-immigrants, however little research exists on Black African American immigrants living in the US (Ade et al., 2011). When referring to obesity, researchers did not notice any significant difference between immigration status and obesity in adult Black African immigrants residing in the US (Ade et al., 2011). Therefore, they found that adult Black African immigrants were not at risk for becoming obese as a result of their immigration standing, but they could be if they consumed too much alcohol (Ade et al., 2011). On the other hand, other researchers found that many West African immigrants who had arrived in the US came with diseases such as obesity and high blood pressure which went undetected in their heritage country (Asgary et al., 2011).

Immigrants who come from developing countries and settle in developed countries tend to modify their lifestyles to that of the local culture of the new dominant society (Regev-Tobias et al., 2012). Being in a new culture shapes the dietary habits and level of physical activity (Ruesch & Volken, 2012). In terms of dietary habits, Black African immigrants living in Canada who maintained the traditional dietary habits of the heritage culture were healthier when they had taken on the dietary habits of the host culture such as with eating nontraditional foods (Delisle, 2010). In fact, when Black African immigrant children maintained close ties to their cultural heritage traditions, they were less likely to become obese and were less likely to obtain sedentary behaviors (Renzaho et al., 2008).

In one study, the caloric intake for Black immigrant children in the US was far less than that of non-immigrant children in the US, but the prevalence of obesity increased for Black African immigrant children as generations continued (Sing et al., 2009). And in a study conducted on Black Bubi immigrants originally from Equatorial Guinea living in Madrid, overall the younger Black Bubi immigrants had a higher tendency to eat Western food as opposed to traditional food (Delisle et al., 2009). However, one third of the participants over 30 years of age chose healthier alternatives such as fruits and vegetables and healthy fats (Delisle et al., 2009). Black Liberian and Somali immigrants consumed 92% of their calories from vegetables upon arrival into the US, whereas only 72% of calories from vegetables were consumed by Americans (Patil et al., 2009). These dietary patterns changed over time in that more calories came from meat, milk, and soda products (Patil et al., 2009). A study in Israel revealed that Black Ethiopian immigrant women, after residing in Israel for more than 14 years, had the same body mass index as native Israeli women, and the Ethiopian women consumed fewer healthier food choices than they did in Ethiopia and consumed more foods higher in simple sugars (Regev-Tobias, Reifen, Endevelt, Havkin, Cohen, Stem, & Stark, 2012). The authors concluded that Ethiopian immigrant women residing in Israel had a higher risk for the development of diseases that resulted from poor eating habits learned from the dominant culture (Regev-Tobias et al., 2012).

Originally, in African nations, obesity has been considered to be healthier than being underweight and obese women have been seen as superior over thin women (Bramble, Cornelius, & Simpson, 2009). However, obesity is now becoming an increasing concern in many developing African nations in that children are taking on poor dietary habits, leading physically inactive lives and becoming obese which can lead to serious health concerns later on in life (Regev-Tobias et al., 2012); Lokuruka, 2013). It is an even greater problem once these immigrants settle into the US or in other countries (Ike-Chinaka, 2013). For example, one researcher examined a sample of Nigerian immigrant children from the ages of 9 to 14 who had lived in the US between 5 to 10 years to determine if they were at a stronger risk for obesity as a result of acculturating (Ike-Chinaka, 2013). The researcher found that the longer Nigerian immigrant children lived in the US, the older they became, and the more at risk they became for obesity. Additionally, the interrelationships between access to fitness facilities and level of socio-economic status to age, body mass, and food selection were significant in diseases including and related to obesity (Ike-Chinaka, 2013).

Summary

In summary, acculturation refers to the processes of cultural change that ensue when an individual interacts with others in another dominant cultural environment (Berry, 1997; Dere et al., 2010). The link between acculturative experiences and health patterns is multifactorial (Helweg-Larsen & Standoff, 2008). Researchers have found that acculturation can have a significant effect on one's physical and mental health (Corral & Landrine, 2008; Zhang & Goodsen, 2011). Acculturative stress is a culmination of psychological and emotional agitation that ensues while one is attempting to acculturate because there is a need for adaptation to more than one culture (Albright et al., 2010). One such form of acculturative stress is perceived discrimination which takes place when a person or people from a group perceive that they are being looked upon critically from others often resulting in having a detrimental effect on the health of those targeted by the discrimination (Hadley et al., 2011). Researchers have also focused on the effects on families during an acculturation experience in that they face many challenges when they resettle into a new country (Renzaho & Vignjevic, 2011). They have also found that acculturation has been associated with risk behaviors such as use of substances, smoking, and alcohol use (Unger et al., 2009).

Resilience, defined as the ability to use protective factors such as positive emotions to adapt to negative circumstances, has been known to assist individuals in reconstructing their identities after tragic events such as war and violence in African nations, and has provided strength in helping them to overcome struggles (Bartholomew, 2012; Greve & Leipold, 2009; Sherwood & Liebling-Kalifani, 2012). It is important to establish resilience in children so that they will grow up to be well-adjusted adults in society (Wu et al., 2013). Furthermore fostering resilience in adolescents is a relevant way to strengthen them psychologically (Lee, Cheung, & Kwong, 2012). For Black African immigrants, resilience has proven to reduce the stress of moving into another country by utilizing resilient behaviors (Obrist & Buchi, 2008).

Obesity has become a global public health problem (CDC, 2009; Stewart-Knox et al., 2012). Obesity rates contribute to unhealthy lifestyle practices such as lack of physical inactivity and poor dietary patterns (Stewart-Knox, et al., 2012). Some of the health risks associated with obesity are, Type 2 diabetes, hypertension, heart disease, osteoarthritis, stroke, and sleep apnea (Aftab et al., 2013; Baranowski et al., 2003; McVeigh, et al., 2013; Turanjanin et al., 2012). Obesity in childhood poses a significant risk for diseases that affect major organs that can eventually lead to morbidity and mortality (Lubans et al., 2010). When children become obese at a young age, they have the potential for becoming obese as adults (Phillips, 2012). It is for this reason that intervention programs such as changing behavior patterns to prevent weight gain in adolescents are effective (Lubans et al., 2010).

Finally, immigrants have also suffered from obesity (Edberg et al., 2011). In general, upon arrival into the host country, immigrants are far less likely to be overweight and obese over their nationally bom counterparts. However, the longer an immigrant lives in the host country, the more chances he or she has of becoming obese (Roshana et al., 2008). In some African nations obesity has been considered to be healthier than being underweight (Bramble et al., 2009). Research studies on Black African immigrants and obesity have been equivocal; for example, researchers did not notice any significant difference between immigration status and obesity in adult Black African immigrants residing in the US (Ade et al., 2011), however, another researcher found that the longer Nigerian immigrant children lived in the US, the more they were at risk for obesity (Ike-Chinaka, 2013).

Chapter 3: Research Method

The problem that was addressed was that the relationships between acculturation, resiliency, obesity health risks, and obesity have not been fully examined in the body of research utilizing the Reserve Capacity Model (RCM: Gallo & Matthews, 2003) specifically for Black African immigrants living in the US. The rate of obesity is 20% for Black African immigrants who currently reside in the US for three years or more (CDC, 2012). The purpose of this study was to examine the influence of acculturation directly and in interaction with resilience on obesity and obesity health risks in a sample of Black African immigrants. The limited research conducted on acculturation, resilience, obesity health risks, and obesity among Black African immigrants has lacked a cohesive theoretical framework, and results from studies on obesity rates in Black African immigrants are equivocal. In accordance with the RCM (Gallo & Matthews, 2003), acculturation and resiliency were likely to play interacting roles to impact Black African immigrants' health risk and health outcomes, including obesity (Venters & Gany, 2011).

The purpose of this quantitative correlational survey research study was to ascertain whether the predictor variable of acculturation was significantly predictive of two criterion variables, obesity health risks and obesity, and whether resilience acted as a moderator between acculturation, obesity health risks, and obesity among Black African immigrants living in the US. In this chapter, the researcher will explain the research questions that were investigated, and the research method and design. Next, the population and sample will be discussed along with the instruments that were used as well as the operational definition of the variables.

For this study, acculturation, the predictor variable, was measured via the Stephenson Multigroup Acculturation Scale (SMAS; Stephenson, 2000). Resilience, the moderating variable, was assessed by the Conner-Davidson Resilience Scale (CD-RISC; Connor & Davidson, 2003). In correspondence with the RCM (Gallo & Matthews, 2003), there were two criterion variables in this study: (a) obesity health risks and (b) obesity. Obesity health risks were assessed by the Weight-Related Symptom Measure (WRSM; Patrick, Bushnell, & Rothman, 2004). The measurement of obesity was a composite scale of three indicators: (a) BMI, (b) waist circumference (in inches), and (c) a single-item used in a national survey (i.e., National Health and Nutrition Examination Survey [NHANES], 2012) inquiring about current perceived weight status. Participants answered the obesity indicators question twice, the first time regarding the current time period, and the second time regarding when they first immigrated to the US. The "past obesity" composite score was entered as a covariate in statistical analysis to remove any associated variance with the criterion variables of obesity risk and obesity: to allow for a purer association between the predictor and criterion variables (Polit, 2010).

In accordance with the RCM (Gallo & Matthews, 2003), the variables of (a) socioeconomic status as the socioeconomic context indicator and (b) the cultural context variables of (a) participant native country, (b) participant native bom status, (c) immigrant generation status, and (d) length of residence in the US were entered as covariates in the statistical analyses. The age and gender of study participants have been associated with obesity risk and obesity in studies with immigrants (Delisle, 2010; Fayombo, 2010; Stewart-Knox et al., 2012) and were also controlled for in the statistical analyses (i.e., were tested as covariates). The following research questions and hypotheses were investigated:

Q1. To what extent, if any, does acculturation, as measured by the SMAS (Stephenson, 2000), predict obesity health risks, as measured by the WRSM (Patrick et al., 2004), in Black African immigrants who currently reside in the US, controlling for study covariates?

Q2. To what extent, if any, does resilience, as measured by the CD-RISC (Connor & Davidson, 2003), moderate between acculturation, as measured by the SMAS (Stephenson, 2000), and obesity health risks, as measured by the WRSM (Patrick et al., 2004), in Black African immigrants who currently reside in the US, controlling for study covariates?

Q3. To what extent, if any, does acculturation, as measured by the SMAS (Stephenson, 2000), predict obesity, as measured by a composite score (i.e., BMI, waist circumference, and perceived current weight status), in Black African immigrants who currently reside in the US, controlling for study covariates?

Q4. To what extent, if any, does resilience, as measured by the CD-RISC (Connor & Davidson, 2003), moderate between acculturation, as measured by the SMAS (Stephenson, 2000), and obesity, as measured by a composite score (i.e., BMI, waist circumference, and perceived current weight status), in Black African immigrants who currently reside in the US, controlling for study covariates?

Hypotheses

Based on the four research questions of this study, four sets of hypotheses are proposed:

Hlo. Acculturation, as measured by the SMAS (Stephenson, 2000) will not significantly predict obesity health risks, as measured by the WRSM (Patrick et al., 2004), in Black African immigrants who currently reside in the US, controlling for study covariates.

H la Acculturation, as measured by the SMAS (Stephenson, 2000) will significantly predict obesity health risks, as measured by the WRSM (Patrick et al., 2004), in Black African immigrants who currently reside in the US, controlling for study covariates.

H2,,. Resilience, as measured by the CD-RISC (Connor & Davidson, 2003), will not significantly moderate between acculturation, as measured by the SMAS (Stephenson, 2000), and obesity health risks, as measured by the WRSM (Patrick et al., 2004), in Black African immigrants who currently reside in the US, controlling for study covariates.

H2a. Resilience, as measured by the CD-RISC (Connor & Davidson, 2003), will significantly moderate between acculturation, as measured by the SMAS (Stephenson, 2000), and obesity health risks, as measured by the WRSM (Patrick et al., 2004), in Black African immigrants who currently reside in the US, controlling for study covariates.

H30. Acculturation, as measured by the SMAS (Stephenson, 2000) will not significantly predict obesity, as measured by a composite score (i.e., BMI, waist circumference, and perceived current weight status), in Black African immigrants who currently reside in the US, controlling for study covariates.

H3*. Acculturation, as measured by the SMAS (Stephenson, 2000) will significantly predict obesity, as measured by a composite score (i.e., BMI, waist circumference, and perceived current weight status), in Black African immigrants who currently reside in the US, controlling for study covariates.

H4o. Resilience, as measured by the CD-RISC (Connor & Davidson, 2003), will not significantly moderate between acculturation, as measured by the SMAS (Stephenson, 2000), and obesity, as measured by a composite score (i.e., BMI, waist circumference, and perceived current weight status), in Black African immigrants who currently reside in the US, controlling for study covariates.

H4». Resilience, as measured by the CD-RISC (Connor & Davidson, 2003), will significantly moderate between acculturation, as measured by the SMAS (Stephenson, 2000), and obesity, as measured by a composite score (i.e., BMI, waist circumference, and perceived current weight status), in Black African immigrants who currently reside in the US, controlling for study covariates.

Research Methods and Design

The proposed study utilized a quantitative correlational survey research design to examine the predictive relationship between acculturation, the predictor (independent) variable, and obesity health risks and obesity, the criterion (dependent) variables; and to determine whether resilience moderated the relationship between acculturation, obesity health risks, and obesity. In the proposed study, a quantitative correlational research design was optimal, as data was gathered from the study participants via self-report measures and statistical tests were conducted to capture the relationships among study phenomena (Kaplan, 2004; Vogt, 2007). A quantitative method was selected due to its preciseness in establishing statistical relationships among numerically-coded variables, allowing for a more objective assessment of the proposed model (Kaplan, 2004; Muijs, 2010). As data in this study are not based on subjective responses of the participants, neither a qualitative nor a mixed method research design was appropriate (Kaplan, 2004; Muijs, 2010). A correlational (survey) research design was necessary as the personal factors measured in this study could not be manipulated by the researcher; in other words, the variables under examination in this study precluded the use of an experimental research design (Vogt, 2007).

Population

According to the Migration Policy Institute (2013), immigrants comprised 38.5 million, or 13% of the total US population in 2011; Black African immigrants comprised 1.48 million or 3.9% of this immigrant population. This population was appropriate to respond to this study's problem and purpose because Black African immigrants were the focus of the study as well as a growing population in the US (Migration Policy Institute, 2013).

Sample

The sample for the study was a convenience sample of 55 Black African immigrants residing in Washington, DC-Baltimore, Maryland area; Boston, Massachusetts, or Chicago, Illinois. In consideration of one primary predictor variable, one moderating variable, and eight covariates, and setting the effect size set at medium, $f^2 = 0.15$, power set at 0.80, the probability level set at $p < 0.05$, the required sample size was 54 (Kelly & Maxwell, 2003). A sample size of 55 participants was planned, as this sample size was large enough to have the power to identify even minimal statistical effects (Kelly & Maxwell, 2003).

The participants were recruited through the Africans' Universe foundation; a community-based foundation located in Boston, Massachusetts that provides outreach and services for African immigrants in the Boston, Massachusetts; Research Chicago, an organization that recruits participants for studies; and Bethel World Outreach, a church located in Silver Springs, Maryland that has a large congregation of African immigrants. The researcher of this study established communication with the Africans' Universe foundation's director, established an agreement with Research Chicago, and established communication with the Executive Director of Bethel Church as the point of contacts who gave the surveys to study participants who met the study sample parameters to invite them to participate in the study. The researcher provided an email link to Africans' Universe and Research Chicago so that the Directors could send it to interested participants containing a consent form that the participant had to sign and a link to the study survey on SurveyMonkey™. Data collection was done via SurveyMonkey™. Participants through Africans' Universe and Research Chicago were sent a SurveyMonkey™ link via their personal email and they completed the survey by clicking on the link. The participants had two months to complete the survey. In order to increase the sample size, the participants were given a chance to win a $100 gift certificate, and were also given $20 to complete the survey.

Materials/Instruments

The predictor variable of acculturation was measured via the Stephenson Multigroup Acculturation Scale (SMAS; Stephenson, 2000). The SMAS has shown to have strong inter-item reliability, with Cronbach's alphas in the high .80s to low .90s (Celenk, & Van de Vijver, 2011; Huynh, Howell, & Benet-Martinez, 2009; Stephenson, 2009). The SMAS has demonstrated sound construct validity, significantly correlating with other measures of acculturation and related constructs, such as familism (Celenk, & Van de Vijver, 2011). The moderating variable of resilience was measured by using the Connor-Davidson Resilience Scale (CD-RISC) (Connor & Davidson, 2003). The CD-RISC has sound inter-item consistency, with Cronbach's alphas in the .80s (Connor & Davidson, 2003). The CD-RISC has been shown to have discriminant validity in determining individuals with and without depression (Ahem, Kiehl, Sole, & Byers, 2006) and has shown to have good construct validity, significantly correlating with other resilience measures (Ahem et al., 2006) and similar constructs such as satisfaction with life (Singh & Yu, 2010). The CD-RISC has been validated in studies with ethnic minority participants (Singh & Yu, 2010). The criterion variable of obesity health risks were assessed by the 20-item Weight-Related Symptom Measure (WRSM: Patrick et al., 2004). The WRSM has shown sound inter-item consistency, with Cronbach's alphas in the .70s, and it has shown good discriminant validity in regard to persons who were and were not obese (Patrick et al., 2004). The criterion variable of obesity status was assessed by three indicators, BMI, waist circumference (in inches), and self-reported perceived weight status, all of which have been validated and used as self-report indicators of obesity (Karasu, 2012; Lin et al., 2012; Rothman, 2008).

Operational Definition of Variables

The primary constructs associated with this proposed research were acculturation, resiliency, obesity health risks, and obesity. There are numerous covariates that were used in the study. The primary variables and covariates are presented below.

Criterion (Independent) Variable/Acculturation. Acculturation refers to the processes of cultural immersion that ensue when an individual interacts and engages with others in the dominant cultural environment (Dere et al., 2010; Stephenson, 2000). The predictor variable of acculturation was measured via the Stephenson Multigroup Acculturation Scale (SMAS; Stephenson, 2000). The questions on the scale refer to the degree to which an individual is immersed into the host culture. Ethnic and cultural behaviors such as language, food, cognition, and interactions are divided into two categories. The Ethnic Society Immersion subscale contains 17 items that measure immersion within one's own culture; example items include "I eat traditional foods from my native culture" and "I think in my native language." The Dominant Society Immersion subscale contains 15 items that assess specific immersion into the American culture. Two examples from this subscale are "I like to eat American foods" and **"I think in English."** The responses for all items are in the form of an interval scale ranging from 1 (false) to 4 (true). The total SMAS score was computed by reverse coding the Ethnic Society Immersion item scores and summing these item scores with item scores on the Dominant Society Immersion scale. The range of scores on the SMAS are 32-128, with higher scores denoting higher levels of acculturation.

Moderating Variable/Resilience. Resilience refers to when one consistently uses positive emotions to adapt to negative circumstances (Greve & Leipold, 2009). The moderating variable of resilience was measured by using the CD-RISC (Connor & Davidson, 2003). The CD-RISC (Connor & Davidson, 2003) consists of 25 items. Respondents answered questions about their attitudes toward adversity; sample items included phrases such as "I stay focused under pressure" and "Coping with stress can strengthen me." The items were scored with a 5-point interval scale, with range of responses coded from (0) not true at all to (4) true nearly all of the time. The score was totaled by summing item scores, with a potential range of scores from 0 to 100; higher scores indicate higher levels of resilience.

Criterion (Dependent) Variable/Obesity Health Risks. Obesity health risks are an indicator of poor health as a result of overweight or obesity (Patrick et al., 2004). The criterion variable of obesity health risks was assessed by the 20-item Weight-Related Symptom Measure (WRSM: Patrick et al., 2004). Participants were asked to rate how much of a problem specific weight-related health conditions were to them using a response scale from 0 (not at all) to 6 (very great deal/bothersome). The types of conditions listed in this survey included (a) frequent urination, (b) increased appetite, (c) shortness of breath, and (d) snoring. The range of scores for the interval-coded WRSM is 0-120, with higher scores denoting higher weight-related symptoms. A score of 80 or higher denotes a greater likelihood of health risk due to obesity.

Criterion (Dependent) Variable/Obesity Status. The measurement of obesity has some inherent issues: (a) oftentimes participants are hesitant to provide actual weight due to the social desirability bias (Karasu, 2012; Lin, Yu, Wu, & Chang, 2012) and (b) the most common assessment of obesity, body mass index (BMI), has some limitations in measurement (e.g., self-report errors, cannot assess muscle mass) (Karasu, 2012; Rothman, 2008). It has been recommended that obesity be assessed via more than one indicator and/or as a composite score (Karasu, 2012). For the purpose of this study, obesity status was assessed by three indicators, all of which have been validated and used as self-report indicators of obesity (Karasu, 2012; Lin et al., 2012; Rothman, 2008).

First, participants were asked their height and weight to determine an interval measure of

BMI, which was calculated by BMI = pounds/(inches)2 X 703 (CDC, 2013). A BMI of

30 or higher indicates obesity (Rothman, 2008). Second, participants were asked their

waist circumference (in inches), an interval measurement (Lin et al., 2012). A waist

circumference of 35 inches for women and 40 inches for men indicates a likelihood of

obesity (Lin et al., 2012). Third, participants were asked to answer a single item, "Do

you consider yourself to be...[currently/when you first came to the United States]" with

responses being overweight (1), underweight (-1), and about the right weight (0). This

item comes from the NHANES (2012).

These three variables were then entered into a principal components analysis

(PCA) with varimax rotation to create composite obesity scores. Studies (e.g., DiStefano,

Zhu, & Mindrila, 2009; Ferrando, 2010; Petersen, Bandeen-Roche, Budtz-Jorgensen, &

Larsen, 2012) have documented that Bartlett scores as composite variables are

psychometrically superior to weighted or standardized scores as well as other types of

factor scores as they are "unbiased estimates of the true factor score" (DiStefano et al.,

2009, p. 4). The Bartlett scores were used as the continuously-coded composite scores of

obesity.

Covariate: Socioeconomic Status. Much research has been devoted to the

appropriate measurement of socioeconomic status, especially among ethnic minority

groups in the US, and results from this research recommend that socioeconomic status be

measured using more than one indicator (Cohen, Doyle, & Baum, 2006; Cowan et al.,

2012; Shavers, 2007). In accordance with measurement best practices (Shavers, 2007)

and in alignment with the RCM (Gall & Matthews, 2003), socioeconomic status was measured as a composite score based on individual and household socioeconomic indicators. Household socioeconomic status was measured via the question, "Which category best depicts your yearly household income before taxes?" (Cohen et al., 2006). This question had six response codes, from 1 (less than $5,000) to 6 (over $100,000).

Individual socioeconomic status was assessed by two questions. The first one was "What is the highest level of education you have attained?" There are five response categories, 1 (no formal education), 2 (high school degree or equivalent), 3 (associate's degree/two-year degree), 4 (bachelor's degree/four-year degree), and 5 (master's degree or higher) (Cowan et al., 2012). The second question was "What is your current employment status?" This item had three response categories, 1 (not currently employed) 2 (employed part-time), and 3 (employed full-time) (Cowan et al., 2012). To develop a composite socioeconomic score that was interval coded, a PCA with varimax rotation was conducted to create Bartlett scores (i.e., unbiased estimates of factor loadings).

Covariate: Native Born Status. The variable of native born status was assessed via a nominal-coded question, "Were you born in the United States?" The response codes are no (0) and yes (1).

Covariate: Native Country. The variable of native country was measured using an open-ended question, "What is your native country?" Participants provided a written response. These responses were transformed into nominally-coded variables (1 = Kenya, 2 = Nigeria ...).

Covariate: Generation Status. The variable of generation status was measured via a nominally-coded question, "What generation of immigrant are you?" with responses of 1 (first generation), 2 (second generation), 3 (third generation), and 4 (fourth generation).

Covariate: Age. Age of participants was obtained by asking participants their age in years. This was an interval-coded variable.

Covariate: Gender. Gender of participants was obtained by asking participants their gender. This variable was a nominal variable where 1 (male) and 2 (female).

Data Collection, Processing, and Analysis

Data was collected via SurveyMonkey™ . Participants from Africans' Universe and Research Chicago were sent a SurveyMonkey™ link via their personal email; they completed the survey by clicking on the link. The participants from Bethel Church were given paper surveys to complete which were distributed to them by the Executive Director of the church. The participants had 2 months to complete the survey. In order to increase the sample size, the participants were given the chance to win a $100 gift card, and were also given $20 to complete the survey.

The researcher conducted hierarchical multiple regression analysis. This type of analysis is utilized when it is necessary to examine the effects of moderation (Aguinis, 1995). Once the data collection period had ended, data was downloaded into an SPSS 21.0 software data file. Prior to conducting hierarchical multiple regression analyses for moderation (Baron & Kenny, 1986; Frazier, Tix, & Barron, 2004), statistical analyses were conducted to gather descriptive information on the sample. The scales were computed and analysis was run for descriptive information on the study variables. Specific statistical tests were conducted to determine and address any violations of assumptions for hierarchical multiple regression (Cohen, 1978; Polit, 2010). The integral assumptions for hierarchical multiple regression analysis were (a) normal distribution of scale scores; (b) reliability of scales; (c) linear associations between the predictor and criterion variable; and (d) homogeneity of variances (homoscedasticity) (Campbell & Campbell, 1983; Polit, 2010).

Normal distributions of data were determined by examining the raw data for outliers and calculating the skewness and kurtosis values. Skewness is an assessment of the degree of symmetry of a distribution of scores: values of $> +/-1.00$ indicate significant violation of a normal distribution of scores (Campbell & Campbell, 1983). Kurtosis indicates the peakedness or flatness of the distribution of scores. The kurtosis value was computed by dividing the kurtosis statistic by the kurtosis standard error (Campbell & Campbell, 1983). If the kurtosis value is $> +/- 2.00$, there is significant peakedness (i.e., the distribution is leptokurtic) or flatness (i.e., the distribution is platykurtic) of the distribution of scores around the mean score (Campbell & Campbell, 1983; Cohen, 1978). Kolmogorov-Smimov Z tests were conducted to test for normality of the distribution of scores (Polit, 2010). The Kolmogorov-Smimov (K-S) Z statistic determines distributional adequacy of scale scores in relation to an assumed population distribution (Polit, 2010). A significant one-sample Kolmogorov-Smimov Z test indicates that the data violate the assumption of normal distribution of scores (Polit, 2010). If data display non-normality, adjustments are made via loglinear transformations (Kaplan, 2004). The reliability of study scales was computed using Cronbach's alphas, with an expectation that alphas should be $> = .70$ (Campbell & Campbell, 1983; Cohen, 1978).

Linear associations between the predictor and criterions variables were assessed via Pearson bivariate correlations. Normal P-P plots and scatterplots were computed to determine normal distribution of data and homoscedasticity (Polit, 2010). The data proves to be linear and show homoscedascity if they are evenly distributed above and below the horizontal line of the scatterplot (Polit, 2010). To ensure that the predictor variable of acculturation did not have variance overlap with the moderating variable of resilience, these variables were examined for collinearity effects via computing a variance inflation factor (VIF) (Polit, 2010). The VIF measures the degree of correlation between beta coefficients and if the VIF value is 5.00 or higher, multicollinearity is evident (Polit, 2010). If multicollineaity was evident, the variables of acculturation and resilience would have been centered (i.e., means computed to zero) and the new centered variables will be used in statistical analyses (Polit, 2010), however multicollinearity was not present.

In this study, a hierarchical multiple regression in accordance with the moderation model proposed by Baron and colleagues (Baron & Kenny, 1986; Frazier, Tix, & Baron, 2004) were utilized. First, the predictor variable of acculturation and the moderating variable of resilience were centered (i.e., mean score is recomputed into 0) and an interaction term (acculturation X resilience) computed (Baron & Kenny, 1986; Frazier et al., 2004). Hierarchical regression analyses were conducted in accordance with moderation (Baron & Kenny, 1986) and guided by the RCM (Gallo & Matthews, 2003): (a) the covariates of past obesity status, age, and gender were entered on the first step of the regression; (b) the covariates of socioeconomic context and the cultural context variables were entered on the second step of the regression; and (c) the un-centered predictor variable of acculturation, the un-centered moderating variable of resilience, and the interaction term (acculturation by resilience) were entered on the third step. If the interaction term is significant, moderation has occurred (Baron & Kenny, 1986; Frazier et al., 2004). This hierarchical regression model was conducted for both criterion variables of obesity risks and obesity. Effect sizes ($f2$) were computed for each hierarchical regression model.

Assumptions

This study was conducted with several assumptions. The assumption of the sample size was considered after the researcher conducted G*Power analysis. The analysis concluded that the required sample size was 54 (Kelly & Maxwell, 2003). However, a sample size of 55 participants was used, as this sample size was large enough to have the power to identify even minimal statistical effects (Kelly & Maxwell, 2003). Another assumption was that the variables have been operationalized correctly. This is because the SMAS (Stephenson, 2000) measuring acculturation, the CD-RISC (Connor & Davidson, 2003) measuring resilience, and the WRSM (Patrick et al., 2004) measuring obesity health risks have all proven to be psychometrically sound with both reliability and validity. Another assumption is that participants gave accurate information regarding their BMI and weight. Prior to conducting statistical analyses for hypothesis testing, descriptive information on the sample was computed. In addition, survey scales were computed and analyses run for descriptive information on study variables. Specific statistical tests were conducted to determine and address any violations of assumptions for hierarchical multiple regression (Cohen, 1978; Polit, 2010). The study hypotheses were tested via hierarchical multiple regression analyses for moderation (Baron & Kenny, 1986; Frazier, Tix, & Barron, 2004).

Limitations

There were limitations to the study. In terms of the study's internal validity, the researcher was not be able to control for the assumption that individuals completing the survey were adults, ages 18 or over, since completing the survey was anonymous. On the other hand, the instruments that were used were not seen as a threat to internal validity since they are psychometrically sound (Cohen & Cohen, 1983; Muijs, 2010). In addition, Black African immigrants who were in the US illegally might have been hesitant to complete a survey for fear of deportation thereby minimizing the potential number of participants. However, this threat was reduced as the researcher collected data through organizations that work with immigrants and had no knowledge as to the study participants' immigrant status. Additionally, some of the questions on the WRSM (Patrick et al., 2004) could have been sensitive in nature, and participants might not have felt comfortable providing information about their weight when calculating their BMI. As a result, while self-reporting their weight, they could have underestimated BMI status due to the embarrassing nature of the questions. This was beyond the control of the researcher.

Delimitations

When referring to delimitations of the study, given that the research was conducted on a sample of Black African immigrants, the researcher chose to focus on only three metropolitan areas in the US—that of the Baltimore/Washington, D.C., Boston, Massachusetts, or Chicago, Illinois. Additionally, the researcher chose to conduct this research on various Black African immigrant ethnicities from various nations, such as Liberia and Kenya for more generalized results, as opposed to being more country specific.

Ethical Assurances

In accordance with the American Psychological Association (2013) researchers must adhere to several ethical standards when conducting research with human subjects. These standards consist of the following: (a) beneficence, or preventing harm; (b) respecting the privacy and dignity of others; (c) accepting responsibility for their actions by obtaining informed consent; and, (d) being honest, truthful, and accurate in all of their applications with psychology.

When referring to beneficence, researchers must take precaution so as to prevent harm to any human subjects at all times. The researcher made sure that the participants were not harmed in any way. In terms of respecting the privacy and dignity of others, the researcher did not collect any personal identifiable data and therefore this did not present itself as a problem. The confidentiality of this information was kept within the confines of the study. When referring to obtaining informed consent, the researcher sought Institutional Review Board (IRB) approval prior to collecting any data. The researcher emailed a letter of consent to the Director of Africans' Universe, to the Executive Director of Bethel church, and to the Director of the Research Chicago recruitment organization to receive their permission to send the survey link to the participants, or give the participants a paper survey for completion. The Director of Africans' Universe, the Executive Director of Bethel Church, and the Director of the Research Chicago recruitment organization were the point persons for sending the survey link to the participants, or giving the participants a paper survey for completion. The participants received a letter of consent upon participating in the study to which they either accepted or did not accept. Finally the researcher practiced honesty, truthfulness, and accuracy when conducting statistical analysis and coding data.

Summary

The purpose of this quantitative correlational survey research study was to ascertain whether the predictor variable of acculturation was significantly predictive of two criterion variables, obesity health risks and obesity, and whether resilience acted as a moderator between acculturation, obesity health risks, and obesity among Black African immigrants living in the US. The construct of acculturation was measured by the SMAS (Stephenson, 2000), the construct of resilience was measured by the CD-RISC (Connor & Davidson, 2003), and obesity health risks were measured by the WRSM (Patrick et al., 2004); all of which were psychometrically sound. Obesity status was measured by a composite measurement of three indicators (self-reported): (a) BMI, (b) waist circumference (in inches), and (c) a single-item as it was used previously in a national survey (i.e., National Health and Nutrition Examination Survey [NHANES], 2012). Prior to conducting statistical analyses for hypothesis testing, descriptive information on the sample was computed. In addition, survey scales were computed and analyses run for descriptive information on study variables. Specific statistical tests were conducted to determine and address any violations of assumptions for hierarchical multiple regression (Cohen, 1978; Polit, 2010). The study hypotheses was tested via hierarchical multiple regression analyses for moderation (Baron & Kenny, 1986; Frazier, Tix, & Barron, 2004).

The limitations of the study consisted of threats to internal validity, including the fact that the researcher was not able to control whether the participants were in fact adults, ages 18 or over, and/or whether the participants provided truthful information on study surveys. Threats to external validity include the lack of the researcher to generalize study findings to specific Black African immigrants (e.g., with regard to birth country and culture). The researcher adhered to the ethical standards as they are outlined in the (2010) American Psychological Association manual, as well as the ethical standards of Northcentral University.

Chapter 4: Findings

Results

The purpose of this quantitative correlational study, using a survey research design, was to ascertain whether the predictor variable of acculturation was significantly predictive of two criterion variables, obesity health risks and obesity, and whether resilience acted as a moderator between acculturation, obesity health risks, and obesity among Black African immigrants living in the US. The researcher conducted the study with 55 participants who were Black African immigrants living in Washington, DC-Baltimore, Maryland area; Boston, Massachusetts, or Chicago, Illinois. Chapter four opens with a presentation of sample demographic, immigration, and weight data results and information. Following discussions on participant demographic, immigration, and weight data is a section devoted to explaining how the obesity composite score was computed as a factor score. The chapter then shifts in focus to present descriptive statistics and scale reliability information of the study variables of acculturation, resilience, obesity health risks, and obesity. Results from statistical testing of study hypotheses are the focus of the next section of the chapter. Substantial attention is then given to the evaluation of the findings with regard to each research question. A summary and interpretation of the research findings conclude the chapter.

Sample Descriptive Statistic Information

The study sample was comprised of 55 Black African immigrants1. All participants resided in the Washington, DC-Baltimore, Maryland area; Boston, Massachusetts; or Chicago Illinois. The sample was comprised of 32 (58.2%) women and 23 (41.8%) men, and the mean age of participants was 38.25 years *(SD* = 13.37). Participants were relatively evenly split between those who were married *(n* = 25, 45.5%) and those who were single *(n* = 30, 54.5%). The majority of participants *(n* = 38, 69.1%) were employed (either full-time or part-time) and were of middle-income status, with the mean income group being $40,000 to $65,000 a year.

The study participants were highly educated, with the majority *(n* = 32, 58.2%) having a bachelor's degree or higher. Results from a chi-square (x^2) goodness of fit test showed that percentage of 58.2% of study participants with bachelor's degrees or higher was significantly higher than the population percentage of 38.0% of Black African immigrants who had bachelor's degrees or higher as reported by Migration Policy Institute researchers (Capps, McCabe, & Fix, 2011), $x^2(1)$ = 4.24, /? = .03. Please see Table 1 for full results.

1The sample was initially N = 56. However, one participant completed less than 30% of the survey and this case was removed from the dataset, resulting in a final N of 55.

Table 1

Study Sample Demographic Descriptive Statistics (N = 55)

	Categories	Frequency	%
Gender			
	Female	32	58.2
	Male	23	41.8
Employment Status			
	Not currently employed	17	30.9
	Employed part-time	10	18.2
	Employed full-time	28	50.9
Marital Status			
	Married	25	45.5
	Single	30	54.5
Household Yearly Income			
	Less than $5,000	2	3.6
	$5,000-$15,000	1	1.8
	$15,000-$40,000	19	34.5
	$40,000-$65,000	20	36.4
	$65,000-$99,999	10	18.2
	Over $99,999	3	4.5
Highest Level of Education			
	No formal education	2	3.6
	High school degree or equivalent	6	10.9

Associate's degree/Two-year degree   15   27.3

Bachelor's degree/Four-year degree   17   30.9

Master's degree or higher   15   27.3

Participants were asked specific questions about their immigration background (see Table 2). The majority of participants $(n = 53, 96.4\%)$ were bom in the US. Of the 55 participants, 25 (45.5 %) were first generation immigrants, 15 (27.3%) were second generation, 8 (14.5%) were third generation, and 7 (12.7%) were fourth generation immigrants. The 55 participants came from 15 African countries, with a higher number of participants being from Liberia $(w = 11, 20.2\%)$, Kenya $(\ll = 10, 18.2\%)$ and Nigeria $\{n = 7, 12.7\%)$.

Table 2

Study Sample Immigrant Descriptive Statistics (N = 55)

	Categories	Frequency	%
Bom in United States			
	Yes	53	96.4
	No	2	3.6
Immigrant Generation Status			
	First generation	25	45.5
	Second generation	15	27.3
	Third generation	8	14.5
	Fourth generation	7	12.7
Native Country			
	Liberia	11	20.2
	Kenya	10	18.2
	Nigeria	7	12.7
	Ghana	6	10.9
	Uganda	5	9.1
	Tanzania	5	9.1
	Niger	2	3.6
	Togo	2	3.6
	Eritrea	1	1.8
	Ethiopia	1	1.8
	South Africa	1	1.8
	Sierra Leone	1	1.8

	Gabon	1	1.8
	Guinea	1	1.8
	Zambia	1	1.8

Table 3 presents descriptive information for participant BMI and waist circumference. Participant BMI ranged from 17.50 to 60.00, with a mean of 28.45 *(SD = 8.68)*. The median BMI was 27.00. The median BMI of 27.00 and the mean BMI of 28.45 demonstrated that these participants were overweight, almost obese, considering that a BMI of 30 is considered obese by the CDC (2013). However, there were six participants with BMIs ranging from 41 to 60; these extreme scores likely inflated the mean BMI value (Cohen, 1978). The waist circumference values ranged from 26.00 to 47.00 inches, with a mean of 34.25 inches *(SD = 5.19)*.

Table 3

Descriptive Statistics for Weight Variables

	N	M	SD	Min	Max	Sk	K	alpha
BMI+	55	28.45	8.68	17.50	60.00	1.82	3.86	N/A
Waist Circumference	55	34.25	5.19	26.00	47.00	.44	-.20	N/A

Note. M = Mean, SD = Standard Deviation, Min = Minimum Score, Max = Maximum Score, Sk = Skewness, K = Kurtosis. +The obesity measure was based on a factor score that combined BMI, waist circumference, and personal perception of weight status.

The 25 participants who were first generation immigrants were asked questions regarding their weight currently and when they first came to America. One (4.0%) participant currently considered him/herself to be underweight, 15 (60.0%) considered themselves to be about the right weight, and 9 (36.0%) considered themselves to be overweight. In contrast, 3 (12.0%) reported that they were underweight, 18 (72.0%)

reported that they were about the right weight, and 4 (16.0%) reported that they were overweight when they immigrated to the US. A chi-square (x2) test of independence was conducted to determine if these 25 participants' perceived current weight status differed from their weight status when they first immigrated to the US. There was a significant difference across past and current perceived weight status groups, $\chi^2(4) = 11.11, p = .025$. There were significantly more participants who reported being underweight *(n = 3)* when they immigrated to the US versus participants who reported that they were currently underweight *(n = 1)*. The 2 participants who stated they were underweight when they first came to America currently reported being about the right weight. Moreover, there were significantly more participants *(n = 9)* who reported currently being overweight as compared to participants (*n = 4*) who reported being overweight when they immigrated to America.

Development of obesity composite score

The obesity composite score was created via a PCA with varimax rotation with the variables of BMI, waist circumference, and perceived current weight status (i.e., underweight, about the right weight, overweight). PCA results showed that these three variables loaded onto one factor, the factor loadings being .66 for perceived current weight, .90 for BMI, and .89 for waist circumference. This one factor had an eigenvalue of 2.02 and explained 67.50% of the variance in the construct of obesity. The Bartlett approach was then conducted; this approach is considered superior to other formulations of factors score as the approach minimizes error variance and maximizes the correlation between the individual factor loadings and the resultant Bartlett factor score (DiStefano et al., 2009; Polit, 2010).

Scale Descriptive Data

The descriptive statistics for the acculturation scale, the resilience scale, the weight-related symptom scale, and the obesity composite score are presented in Table 4.

Table 4

Descriptive Statistics for Study Variables

	N	M	SD	Min	Max	Sk	K	alpha
Acculturation	55	78.05	18.60	40.00	11700	-.25	-.43	.92
Resilience	55	70.71	19.39	31.00	100.00	-.48	-.77	.95
Weight-Related Symptoms	55	19.85	17.94	0.00	68.00	.77	.63	.85
Obesity+	55	0.00	1.00	-1.31	2.85	1.06	.78	N/A

Note. M = Mean, SD = Standard Deviation, Min = Minimum Score, Max = Maximum Score, Sk = Skewness, K = Kurtosis.+ The obesity value is a composite Bartlett factor score that combined BMI, waist circumference, and personal opinion of weight status.

Testing of assumptions. The scales were examined for inter-item reliability by conducting Cronbach's alpha. The scales of acculturation, resilience, and weight-related health symptoms had Cronbach's alphas of .92, .95, and .85, respectively. As a Cronbach's alpha of >= .70 is considered adequate, these are considered good to excellent inter-item reliabilities (Cohen, 1978).

The scales were then examined to determine whether they violated the assumption of normality. None of the variables had skewness or kurtosis values of >= 2.00, which showed that they were normally distributed (Campbell & Campbell, 1983; Cohen, 1978). Normal distribution was further validated by the normal P-P plots of scales, as was homoscedasticity (see Figures 2 - 5).

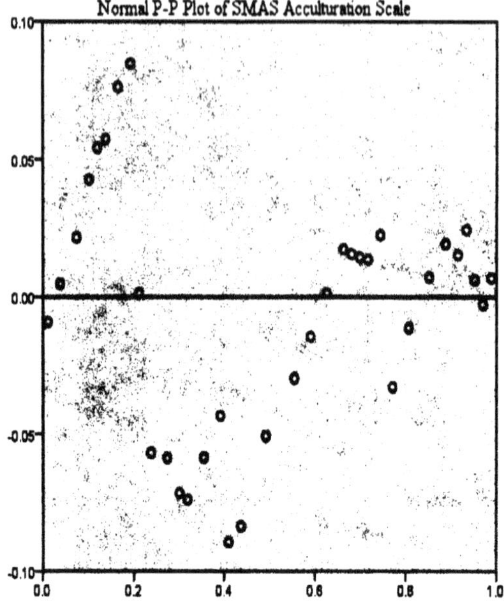

Figure 2. Normal P-P plot of acculturation scale

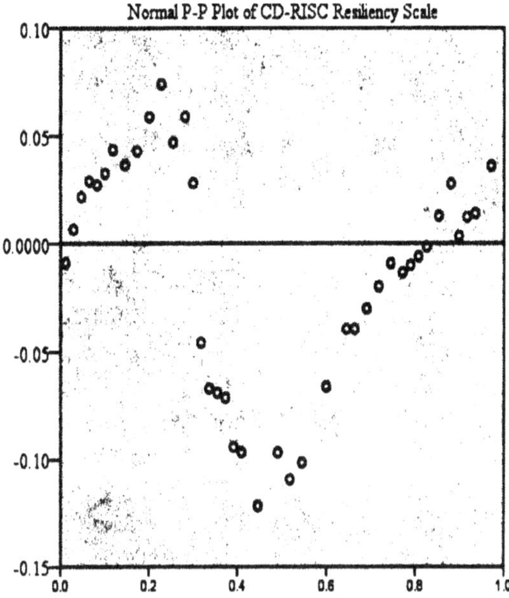

Figure 3. Normal P-P plot of resilience scale

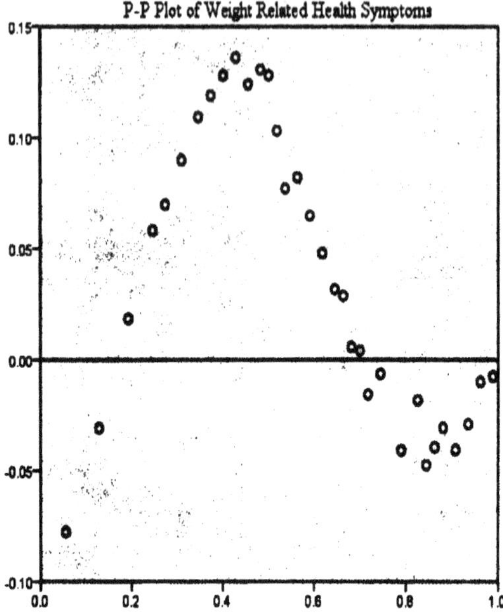

Figure 4. Normal P-P plot of weight-related health symptoms scale

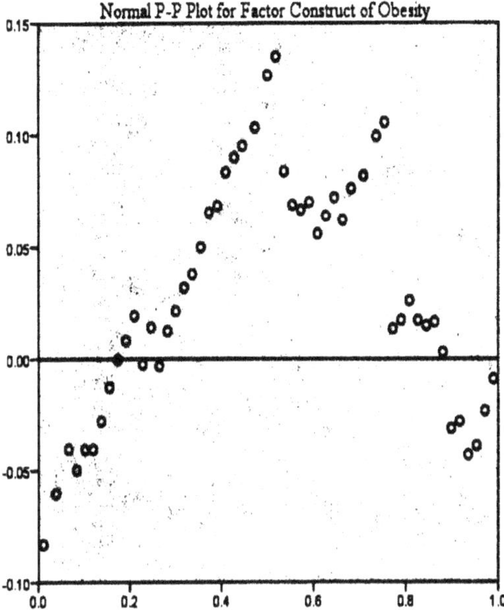

Figure 5. Normal P-P plot of obesity scale

Pearson bivariate correlations. Two series of Pearson bivariate correlations were conducted. The first Pearson bivariate correlation was conducted between the acculturation and resilience variables to determine whether the assumption of lack of multicollinearity was met. Acculturation was significantly correlated with resilience, $r(55) = .30, p = .025$, but not at the $r >= .80$ level required for multicollinearity (Polit, 2010). The variance inflation factor (VIF) value of 1.00 further validated the lack of multicollinearity between acculturation and resilience (Polit, 2010).

The second series of Pearson bivariate correlations were conducted with the demographic and immigration variables and the study variables of acculturation, resilience, weight-related health symptoms, and obesity (see Table 5). Results showed that the demographic variables of gender, marital status, yearly household income, and employment status were not significantly associated with acculturation, resilience, obesity health risks, or obesity. These variables were not entered as covariates in the hierarchical multiple linear regression analyses for hypothesis testing. The variables that were significant with at least one study variable—and thus were covariates— were the demographic variables of age and highest level of education, the immigration variables of having been bom in the US, immigrant generation status, and their native African country, and the weight-related variable of participants' perceived weight status when they immigrated to the US. Taken one step further, age was significantly correlated with resilience, highest level of education was significantly correlated with resilience, having been bom in the US was significantly correlated with resilience, immigrant generation status was significantly correlated with acculturation, obesity health risks, and obesity, and finally, native African Country was significantly correlated with obesity.

Table 5

Pearson Bivariate Correlations: Demographic and Immigrant Variables and the Study Variables of Acculturation, Resilience, Weight-Related Health Symptoms, and Obesity (N = 55)

	Acculturation	Resilience	Weight-Related Health Symptoms	Obesity
Age	.50***	.09	.30*	.42**
Gender	-.11	-.15	.21	.13
Marital Status	.23	.03	-.11	-.19
Yearly Household Income	-.19	-.10	.02	-05
Employment Status	-.01	.23	-.06	.15
Highest Level of Education	.08	.29*	-.04	.11
Bom in United States	.14	.30*	-.17	.09
Immigrant Generation Status	.29*	.13	-.29*	-.32*
Native African Country	.12	-.07	-.05	-.32*

Note. $*p < .05$; $**p < .01$; $***p < .001$.

Data Analyses for Hypothesis Testing

A hierarchical multiple linear regression for moderation (Baron & Kenny, 1986) was conducted to address the first two research questions. The hierarchical multiple linear regression for moderation analysis was conducted with specific steps, resulting in two models (Baron & Kenny, 1986). The first regression model contained the five covariates of age, highest level of education, being bom in the US, immigrant generation status, and native African country. All of these variables were entered at the first step of the hierarchical multiple linear regression for moderation. The second regression model contained the variables of acculturation and resilience and the interaction term of acculturation by resilience used to test for moderation effects. These three variables were entered at the second step of the hierarchical multiple linear regression for moderation.

The dependent variable was weight-related health symptoms.

Table 6 provides results from the hierarchical multiple linear regression for moderation. The results showed that the first model comprised of the five covariates was not significant, $F(5,47) = 1.78$, $p = .136$, $R2 = .159$. When examining univariate effects, there were no significant predictors of weight-related health symptoms.

The second model, comprised of the five covariates and the variables of acculturation, resilience, and the interaction term of acculturation by resilience was significant, $F(3,44) = 11.18$, $p < .001$. Based on the R2 change of .364, the new variables in the model collectively explained an additional 36.4% of the variance in weight-related health symptoms. That is, the variables that made this model significant were acculturation, resilience, and the acculturation by resilience interaction term. Acculturation significantly predicted weight-related health symptoms, $P = -.297$, $p = 043$. Based on the coding of variables, *higher* levels of acculturation predicted *fewer* weight-related health symptoms. Resilience significantly predicted weight-related health symptoms, $3 = -.518$, $p < .001$. The results showed that *higher* levels of resilience were associated with *fewer* weight-related health symptoms. Resilience also significantly moderated between acculturation and weight-related health symptoms, $p = -.311$, $p = .011$. The results showed that high levels of resilience were associated with the fewest weight-related health symptoms when the participant also had high acculturation levels.

Table 6

Hierarchical Multiple Linear Regression: Age, Highest Level of Education, Born in United States, Immigrant Generation Status, Native African Country, Acculturation, Resilience, and the Interaction of Acculturation and Resilience on Weight-Related Health Symptoms (N = 55)

	B	T	R	R2	SEE	R²change	F	df	/T"
Model 1			399	359	1734	359	L78	5Al	A36
Age	304	1.77							.083
Highest Level of Education	-.162	-1.11							.273
Bom in United States	-.184	-1.31							.196
Immigrant Gen Status	-.103	-0.63							.530
Native African Country	-.059	-0.43							.669
Model 2			.723	.523	13.50	.364	11.18	3,44	<.001
Age	.230	1.50							.141
Highest Level of Education	.064	0.52							.605
Bom in United States	.039	0.33							.740
Immigrant Gen Status	-.011	-0.08							.934
Native African Countiy	-.045	-0.42							.674
Acculturation	-.297	-2.08							.043
Resilience	-.518	-4.28							<.001
Acculturation X Resilience	-.311	-2.66							.011

A hierarchical multiple linear regression for moderation (Baron & Kenny, 1986) was conducted to address the last two research questions. The first model of the hierarchical multiple linear regression analysis contained the covariates of age, highest level of education, being born in the US, immigrant generation status, and native African country. All of these variables were entered at the first step of the hierarchical multiple linear regression for moderation. The second model contained the variables of acculturation and resilience and the interaction term of acculturation by resilience. These three variables were entered at the second step of the hierarchical multiple linear regression for moderation. The dependent variable was obesity.

The results showed that the first model, comprised of the six covariates was significant, $F(5,47) = 3.01$ $p = .019$. Based on the model R2 of .243, this model explained 24.3% of the variance in the outcome of obesity. However, when examining individual predictive effects, there were no significant individual predictors. As such, these variables collectively predicted obesity.

The second model, comprised of the covariates and the variables of acculturation, resilience, and the interaction term of acculturation by resilience was not significant, $F(3,44) = 0.92, p = .441$. There were no significant individual predictor effects of acculturation, resilience, and the interaction of acculturation by resilience. Despite this lack of significance, the addition of the acculturation, resilience, and the acculturation by resilience term variables collectively explained an additional 4.5% of the variance in obesity, based on the R change of .045.

Table 7

Hierarchical Multiple Linear Regression: Age, Highest Level of Education, Born in United States, Immigrant Generation Status, Native African Country, Acculturation, Resilience, and The Interaction of Acculturation and Resilience on Obesity (N = 55)

	5	f							
Model 1			492	243	092	243	101	547	XH9
Age	290	1.78							.082
Highest Level of Education	-.039	-0.28							.782
Bom in United States	.094	0.70							.485
Immigrant Gen Status	-.208	-1.35							.185
Native African Country	-.194	-1.49							.144
Model 2			.536	.287	0.93	.045	0.92	3,44	.441
Age	.227	1.21							.233
Highest Level of Education	.048	0.32							.750
Bom in United States	.158	1.12							.270
Immigrant Gen Status	-.185	-1.18							.244
Native African Country	-.190	-1.45							.153
Acculturation	-.110	-0.63							.531
Resilience	-.175	-1.18							.244
Acculturation X Resilience	.027	0.19							.852

Evaluation of Findings

The theoretical framework that guided this study was Gallo and Matthews' (2003) Reserve Capacity Model (RCM), a model that was derived from the acculturation theory (Berry, 1997) and Social Cognitive Theory (SCT; Bandura, 2011). The RCM (Gallo & Matthews, 2003) posited that the sociocultural factors, consisting of either socioeconomic status and/or cultural contexts, inclusive of acculturation, interact with reserve capacity resources, such as personal resilience to influence both health risks and health outcomes in immigrants. In the current study, the social context was represented by acculturation, the reserve capacity resource was represented by personal resilience, and the health risks and outcomes were represented by obesity health risks and obesity. Consistent with predictions made by the RCM, the results showed that high levels of personal resilience were associated with the fewest weight-related health symptoms when the participant also had higher acculturation levels which correctly correlates with the RCM. On the other hand, contrary to the predictions made by the RCM, acculturation, as it interacted with personal resilience did not have an effect on health outcomes in immigrants. Furthermore, higher levels of acculturation alone had a positive impact on minimizing health risks, also contrary to the RCM because resilience was not used as a reserve capacity resource. The current study was different from other studies that have been guided by the RCM in that prior studies did not focus specifically on acculturation as it relates to resilience, obesity health risks, and obesity.

Gallo et al (2005) conducted a study guided by the RCM on primarily White middle-aged women and found that, as predicted by the RCM, women with lower levels of socioeconomic status (the sociocultural context) had fewer personal resilience reserves (the reserve capacity resource) and therefore produced more emotional reactions (the health risk) which led to stress (the outcome). And Matthews, Raikkonen, Gallo, and Kuller (2008) conducted a study guided by the RCM on primarily White women regarding metabolic syndrome. Consistent with the RCM, the authors found that, lower levels of socioeconomic status (the sociocultural context) led to lower levels of personal resilience (the reserve resource capacity) which led to more instances of negative emotions (the health risk) and then metabolic syndrome (the outcome) (Matthews et al., 2008). All in all, it is important to note that in both studies conducted by Gallo et al (2005) and Matthews et al (2008), the authors utilized a White population, but in the current study, a sample of Black African immigrants was used, which is unprecedented. Therefore, the current study is the first study to examine the Black African immigrant population through the RCM theoretical framework.

When discussing the hypotheses, the null hypothesis HIo for the first research question was, "Acculturation, as measured by the SMAS (Stephenson, 2000) will not significantly predict obesity health risks, as measured by the WRSM (Patrick et al., 2004), in Black African immigrants who currently reside in the US, controlling for study covariates." Acculturation did significantly predict obesity health risks based on the statistical outcome of $f/?(55) = -.297$, $p=.04$, and therefore the researcher rejected the null hypothesis. On the other hand, the statistical outcome was also opposite of the alternate hypothesis. The higher score on the acculturation score means higher levels of acculturation and a higher score on obesity health risks means more symptoms. Therefore, the result can be interpreted that higher levels of acculturation were related to fewer symptoms. Consequently, overall, the results showed that in general, *higher* levels of acculturation were associated with *fewer* obesity health risks. This contradicts other studies on acculturation and obesity health risks. For example, Regev-Tobias et al (2012) conducted a study on Black African Ethiopian women who had acculturated in Israel for more than 7 years. The authors found that the women had an increase in body mass, and consumed more foods high in sugar and fewer healthy foods such as fruits and vegetables, concluding that these women faced a much higher risk for obesity related diseases as a result of acculturating to a developed country. Therefore higher levels of acculturation were associated with more weight-related health symptoms, which is different from the results of the current study.

The null hypothesis H2o for the second research question was, "Resilience, as measured by the CD-RISC (Connor & Davidson, 2003), will not significantly moderate between acculturation, as measured by the SMAS (Stephenson, 2000), and obesity health risks, as measured by the WRSM (Patrick et al., 2004), in Black African immigrants who currently reside in the US, controlling for study covariates." Resilience did not significantly moderate between acculturation and obesity health risks based on the statistical outcome of $/?(55) = -.311$, p=.011., and therefore the researcher failed to reject the null hypothesis. On the other hand, the statistical outcome was also *opposite* of the alternate hypothesis. Overall, the results showed that higher levels of resilience were associated with the fewest obesity health risks when the participant also had high acculturation levels. The findings on resilience and acculturation in the current study agree with former studies that were conducted on African immigrants, however there were no other studies on acculturation, resilience, and obesity health risks. In one study however, Obrist and Buchi (2008) concluded that resilience proved to reduce the stress of moving into another country by utilizing resilient behaviors and resilience moderated acculturation. In another study, Kamya (1997) found that spiritual well-being had a positive correlation with resilience as coping mechanisms for dealing with acculturative stress in the host culture for Black African immigrants in the US. Therefore, in both studies conducted by Obrist and Buchi (2008) and Kamya (1997), resilience moderated the effects of acculturation.

The null hypothesis H3o for the third research question was, "Acculturation, as measured by the SMAS (Stephenson, 2000) will not significantly predict obesity, as measured by a composite score (i.e., BMI, waist circumference, and perceived current weight status), in Black African immigrants who currently reside in the US controlling for study covariates. There were no significant individual predictor effects of acculturation since $/?(55) = -.110$, $p = .531$ in predicting obesity, and therefore, the researcher failed to reject the null hypothesis. This contradicts other studies that have been conducted on acculturation and obesity. For example, in one study, the authors found that the further African immigrants moved away from the traditional foods they once consumed as soon as they acculturated into the new culture, the more likely they consumed foods that led to obesity, and they became less physically active (Renzaho et al., 2008). Additionally, Ike-Chinaka (2013) examined a sample of Nigerian immigrant children who had lived in the US between 5 and 10 years and determined that they were at a higher risk for obesity as a result of acculturating. The author also found that the longer immigrant children lived in the US and the older they became they were more at risk for obesity. Therefore, higher levels of acculturation were positively associated with obesity which is opposite of the findings in the current study; acculturation was not positively associated with obesity.

Finally, the null hypothesis of H4o for the fourth question was, "Resilience, as measured by the CD-RISC (Connor & Davidson, 2003), will not significantly moderate between acculturation, as measured by the SMAS (Stephenson, 2000), and obesity, as measured by a composite score (i.e., BMI, waist circumference, and perceived current weight status), in Black African immigrants who currently reside in the US controlling for study covariates." When comprising the covariates and the variables of acculturation, resilience, and the interaction term of acculturation by resilience, there was no significance, $/?(55) = .027, p = .825$. Therefore the researcher failed to reject the null hypothesis. The findings on resilience and acculturation in the current study disagree with former studies that were conducted on African immigrants however there were no other studies on acculturation, resilience, and obesity. In one study on Somali adolescent immigrants in the US, researchers found that spiritual beliefs and mental health counseling led to higher levels of resilience which ameliorated the side effects of acculturative stress upon arrival into the new country Ellis et al (2010). In another study on Black African immigrants in Switzerland, these immigrants experienced more stress upon arrival in the new country while acculturating however they were able to adjust during the acculturation experience by developing life skills that enabled them to master the stress with the use of resilient behaviors (Obrist & Buchi, 2008). Therefore, in both studies conducted by Obrist and Buchi (2008) and Ellis et al (2010) resilience moderated the effects of acculturation.

One rationale could be that individuals who are obese may have a high self-esteem whether they are obese and therefore do not feel the need to rely on resilience to prevent obesity. Another reason could be that these individuals have more significant concerns over being obese or becoming obese. For example, they could use their inner resilience to maintain and strengthen other areas in their lives other than their weight, such as education, work, or social networks.

The RCM posited that the sociocultural factors of socioeconomic status and the cultural context, inclusive of acculturation, interact with personal resilience, to influence both health risks and health outcomes in immigrants. The RCM was consistent in predicting that high levels of personal resilience were associated with the fewest obesity health risks when the participant also had high acculturation levels. On the other hand, the RCM was inconsistent in predicting that acculturation, as it interacted with personal resilience did not have an effect on health outcomes in immigrants. Higher levels of acculturation alone had a positive impact on minimizing health risks, not resilience, also inconsistent with the RCM.

Summary

In summary, this study was designed to ascertain whether the predictor variable of acculturation was significantly predictive of two criterion variables, obesity health risks and obesity, and whether resilience acted as a moderator between acculturation, obesity health risks, and obesity among Black African immigrants living in the US. Of the 55 study participants, 32 (58.2%) were female and 23 (41.8%) were male; the mean age of participants was 38.25 years. All in all, higher levels of acculturation were associated with fewer obesity health risks. Higher levels of resilience were associated with the fewest obesity health risks when the participants also had high acculturation levels. Finally, acculturation did not significantly predict obesity and resilience did not significantly moderate between acculturation and obesity for Black African immigrants.

Chapter 5: Implications, Recommendations, and Conclusions

Despite previous research utilizing the RCM as a framework (Gallo & Matthews, 2003; Gallo et al., 2009), until now, no researchers have ever examined the constructs of acculturation, resilience, obesity health risks, and obesity on a sample of Black African immigrants, and therefore this study is unique. The problem that was addressed in this study is that the relationships between acculturation, resiliency, obesity health risks, and obesity have not been fully examined in the body of research utilizing the Reserve Capacity Model (RCM: Gallo & Matthews, 2003) specifically for Black African immigrants living in the US. The purpose of this quantitative correlational survey research study was to ascertain whether the predictor variable of acculturation was significantly predictive of two criterion variables, obesity health risks and obesity, and whether resilience acted as a moderator between acculturation, obesity health risks, and obesity among Black African immigrants living in the US. The researcher utilized a quantitative correlational survey research design to examine the predictive relationship between acculturation, the predictor (independent) variable, and obesity health risks and obesity, the criterion (dependent) variables; and to determine whether resilience moderated the relationship between acculturation, obesity health risks, and obesity.

The construct of acculturation was measured by the SMAS (Stephenson, 2000), the construct of resilience was measured by the CD-RISC (Connor & Davidson, 2003), and obesity health risks was measured by the WRSM (Patrick et al., 2004); all of which were psychometrically sound. Obesity status was measured by a composite measurement of three indicators (self-reported): (a) BMI, (b) waist circumference (in inches), and (c) a single-item as it was used previously in a national survey (i.e., National Health and

Nutrition Examination Survey [NHANES], 2012). Prior to conducting statistical analyses for hypothesis testing, descriptive information on the sample was computed. In addition, survey scales were computed and analyses run for descriptive information on study variables. Specific statistical tests were conducted to determine and address any violations of assumptions for hierarchical multiple regression (Cohen, 1978; Polit, 2010). The study hypotheses were tested via hierarchical multiple regression analyses for moderation (Baron & Kenny, 1986; Frazier, Tix, & Barron, 2004).

There were several limitations to the study. In terms of the study's internal validity, the researcher was not be able to control for the assumption that individuals completing the survey were adults, ages 18 or over, since completing the survey was anonymous. On the other hand, the instruments that were used were not seen as a threat to the internal validity since they are psychometrically sound (Cohen & Cohen, 1983; Muijs, 2010). In addition, Black African immigrants who were in the US illegally might have been hesitant to complete a survey for fear of deportation thereby minimizing the potential number of participants. However, this threat was reduced as the researcher collected data through organizations that worked with immigrants and had no knowledge as to the study participants' immigrant status. Additionally, some of the questions on the WRSM (Patrick et al., 2004) could have been sensitive in nature, and participants might not have felt comfortable providing information about their weight when calculating their BMI. As a result, while self-reporting their weight, they could have underestimated their BMI status due to the embarrassing nature of the questions. This was beyond the control of the researcher.

There were also limitations of the study as it relates to the external validity. External validity is defined as the capability to make results generalized amongst various groups of people or scenarios (Cohen & Cohen, 1983; Muijs, 2010). One threat to the external validity was that the researcher had focused on Black African immigrants, but not on a specific ethnicity within the Black African immigrant population. Therefore, results could have been overly generalized to describe all Black African immigrant populations despite the country or culture from which they came.

This study was conducted in an ethical manner and in accordance with the standards set forth by the American Psychological Association (2013). The researcher prevented harm from participants, respected their privacy and dignity, accepted responsibility by obtaining informed consent from each of the participants before conducting the study, and was honest, truthful, and accurate in all applications of psychology. The researcher received approval to conduct this study by Northcentral University's IRB prior to collecting data. The researcher did not collect any personal identifiable data, and confidentiality of the data that was collected was kept within the confines of the study.

This chapter will begin with the implications of the study as they pertain to each individual hypothesis and contribute to the existing literature, as well as any limitations that could have affected the interpretation of the findings of the study. Next, the researcher will describe how the results respond to the study problem, fit with the purpose of the study, and demonstrate significance.

Implications

For this study, the focus was to determine whether the predictor variable of acculturation was significantly predictive of two criterion variables, obesity health risks and obesity, and whether resilience acted as a moderator between acculturation, obesity health risks, and obesity among Black African immigrants living in the US. Implications from prior research have concluded that higher levels of acculturation have led to more obesity and obesity health risks (Ike-Chinaka, 2013; Renzaho et al., 2008) which is different from the results of this study. On the other hand, prior research has concluded that resilience ameliorates the negative side effects of acculturation (Kamya, 1997; Obrist & Buchi, 2008) which was a similar finding in this study because higher levels of acculturation were associated with fewer obesity health risks when participants had higher levels of acculturation.

There are some possible justifications with regard to the differences between the results from this study in comparison to the results from prior studies. Research question 1 was, "To what extent, if any, does acculturation, as measured by the SMAS (Stephenson, 2000), predict obesity health risks, as measured by the WRSM (Patrick et al., 2004), in Black African immigrants who currently reside in the US, controlling for study covariates?" While higher levels of acculturation have led to obesity and obesity health risks in prior studies (Ike-Chinaka, 2013; Renzaho et al., 2008) as mentioned previously, the results from this study were significantly different, because higher levels of acculturation were associated with fewer obesity health risks. One explanation could be that the participants were highly educated and also had high levels of socioeconomic status. This could mean that the higher the level of education and the higher the level of socioeconomic status an individual possesses, the less likely he or she will become obese as a result of an acculturation experience. For example, the participants could have been educated in the areas of health and physical fitness which could have equipped them with the knowledge on how to choose healthier foods over unhealthier foods, and to exercise more to keep the weight off. Or, they could have afforded more expensive food options that were healthier, thereby preventing health risks. Another explanation could be that these participants were more fluent in the English language and were better able to communicate and therefore had better access to healthcare. Since not all immigrants are able to speak the English language fluently, when they arrive in a new country they come up against many barriers such as lack of medical care and poverty (Harawa, Bingham, Cichran, Greenland, & Cunningham, 2002). One limitation that could have affected the interpretation of the results is that the focus was on Black African immigrants in general, not on a specific ethnicity within Black African immigrant populations. Therefore, results could have been overly generalized to describe all Black African immigrant populations despite the country or culture and socioeconomic level from which they came.

Research question 2 was, "To what extent, if any, does resilience, as measured by the CD-RISC (Connor & Davidson, 2003), moderate between acculturation, as measured by the SMAS (Stephenson, 2000), and obesity health risks, as measured by the WRSM (Patrick et al., 2004), in Black African immigrants who currently reside in the US, controlling for study covariates?" The results indicated that higher levels of resilience were associated with the fewest obesity health risks when the participant also had high acculturation levels. The possible explanation could be that the more resilience an individual possesses, the less he or she is affected by acculturation stressors. The higher the level of acculturation could mean that individuals are better assimilated into the new culture, and therefore, obesity health risks are minimized. This is a significant finding in that the leaders of immigration organizations and medical practitioners can learn and understand that resilience ameliorates acculturation experiences. Therefore, it minimizes stress. The more immigrant organizations and medical practitioners can incorporate resilience programs and training into immigrant communities, health problems associated with obesity can be prevented, or ameliorated. As a result, there will be less reliance on healthcare and in turn, governmental organizations of the federal, state, and local levels will realize financial savings in their programs. One limitation that could have affected the interpretation of the results is that participants might have felt uncomfortable completing some of the questions on the WRSM (Patrick et al., 2004) scale. Therefore, they might not have been truthful in their responses.

For Q3, the results were not significant in determining, "To what extent, if any, does acculturation, as measured by the SMAS (Stephenson, 2000), predict obesity, as measured by a composite score (i.e., BMI, waist circumference, and perceived current weight status), in Black African immigrants who currently reside in the US, controlling for study covariates? One explanation could be that the *perception* of weight was misconstrued in that participants could have perceived that they did not become obese while acculturating in the US. Therefore, it is not known if immigrants' weight was the true weight that they indicated. Another explanation could be that higher levels of education prevented them from becoming obese. As mentioned earlier, they could have been educated in the areas of health and physical fitness which equipped them with the knowledge on how to choose healthier foods over unhealthier foods and exercising more to keep the weight off. In addition, earning higher salaries could have afforded them with the luxury of purchasing healthier foods which tend to cost more over foods that are higher in sugar and fat. It has been noted that among the factors that lead to obesity are lack of physical activity, poor dietary patterns, over consumption of foods high in fat and carbohydrates, and urbanization (Lokuruka, 2013). The point regarding earning a higher salary is consistent with Ike-Chinaka's acculturation study (2013) in that possessing a lower level of socio-economic status was significant in obtaining diseases including and related to obesity (Ike-Chinaka, 2013). One limitation that could have affected the interpretation of the results is that participants might not have felt comfortable providing information about their weight when calculating their BMI. As a result, while self-reporting their weight, they could have underestimated or overestimated their BMI status due to the embarrassing nature of the question, or based on their own inaccurate perceptions of their weight.

For Q4, the results were not significant in determining the question, "To what extent, if any, does resilience, as measured by the CD-RISC (Connor & Davidson, 2003), moderate between acculturation, as measured by the SMAS (Stephenson, 2000), and obesity, as measured by a composite score (i.e., BMI, waist circumference, and perceived current weight status), in Black African immigrants who currently reside in the US, controlling for study covariates?" Resilience did not moderate between acculturation and obesity. One logical explanation could be that individuals who were already overweight and acculturated did not necessarily need to rely on resilience to prevent them from becoming obese. Previous authors have examined resilience in relation to acculturation, but not with obesity. With regard to acculturation and obesity, the findings from one study concluded that if Black African immigrants were obese upon arrival in the host country during an acculturation experience, they were more at risk to remain obese throughout their stay (Hervey, Vargas, Klesges, Fischer, Trippel, & Juhn, 2009). That being said, the immigrants in the current study who were already obese prior to migrating to the US might not have relied on resilience to control their weight. Perhaps they had higher self-esteem levels and therefore did not need to rely on resilience to prevent obesity or be affected by it. Another reason could be that these individuals are less concerned with being obese or becoming obese and more concerned with other areas of their lives, such as family, education, maintaining employment, and establishing strong social networks. They could also be utilizing their inner resilience to maintain and strengthen those other areas of their lives. On the other hand, these immigrants could have already been resilient because of the strong social support systems they had already established with family members. This is because, family and the presence of a familiar ethnic community enables immigrants to feel included and provides them with access to the larger society (Simich, Beiser, Stewart, & Mwakarimba, 2005).

One limitation that could have skewed the results of this question is that more than half of the participants came from a church and had strong spiritual beliefs. Researchers have found that Africans, in general, gain strength through strong spiritual beliefs, and their philosophy of life is expressed through prayer and praises (Finley & Alexander, 2009). That being said, those participants with strong spiritual beliefs could have made the results on resilience much more significant as opposed to having participants with none to minimal spiritual beliefs.

The results of the study responded to the study problem which was that the relationships between acculturation, resiliency, obesity health risks, and obesity have not been fully examined in the body of research utilizing the Reserve Capacity Model (RCM: Gallo & Matthews, 2003) specifically for Black African immigrants living in the US. This is the first study of its kind incorporating the RCM as a guiding framework for a sample of Black African immigrants. The results also correspond with the purpose of this quantitative correlational survey research study which was to ascertain whether the predictor variable of acculturation was significantly predictive of two criterion variables, obesity health risks and obesity, and whether resilience acted as a moderator between acculturation, obesity health risks, and obesity among Black African immigrants living in the US. Higher levels of acculturation were associated with fewer obesity health risks. Higher levels of resilience were associated with fewer obesity health risk symptoms when the participant also had high acculturation levels. Additional results showed that neither acculturation nor resilience significantly predicted obesity, respectively. The most significant contribution of this study is its examination of acculturation, resilience, obesity health risks, and obesity outcomes among Black African immigrants using Gallo and Matthew's (2003) RCM theoretical framework.

Recommendations

The results of this study are extremely relevant to Black African immigrant communities. There are many practical ways that the findings from this research can be applied to Black African immigrant communities. This study has shown that resilience significantly predicted fewer obesity health risks, and moderated between acculturation and obesity health risk symptoms. It has also allowed for a new understanding of the interactions between acculturation, resilience, obesity health risks, and obesity for Black

African immigrants. It is because of this new understanding that leaders of mental health and healthcare organizations can serve Black African immigrants in a more meaningful way. They can establish programs that will help to build resilience in immigrants so that obesity health risks can be prevented. Leaders can establish additional education in obesity prevention programs to address those factors of acculturation and resilience that play a role in obesity and obesity health risks. Education may play a key role in preventing obesity and obesity health risks for the future. Results from this study will also help to promote health initiatives in Black African immigrant communities to link individuals to needed healthcare services.

This study also has numerous theoretical and research contributions. This study has contributed to acculturation and resilience theories by providing a better understanding of how acculturation and resiliency processes influence health outcomes in Black African immigrants. Perhaps the most significant contribution of this study is its examination of acculturation, resilience, obesity health risks, and obesity outcomes among Black African immigrants using Gallo and Matthew's (2003) RCM theoretical framework. To date, the RCM framework (Gallo & Matthews, 2003) has never been tested on a sample of Black African immigrants. Finally, this study is important with regard to its contribution to the minimal body of research that has assessed obesity rates in Black African immigrants (e.g., Ade et al., 2011; Asgary et al., 2011). While the study did not provide national rates of obesity among Black African immigrants, it provided obesity and obesity health risk data on Black African immigrant samples in specific US communities. For future studies, researchers could examine obesity and obesity health risks over time in relation to the constructs of acculturation and resilience. It is also recommended that future research include the examination of other cultural factors, such as the individual's native country, that may be associated with obesity and health risks related to obesity.

Conclusions

This study examined whether the predictor variable of acculturation was significantly predictive of two criterion variables, obesity health risks and obesity, and whether resilience acted as a moderator between acculturation, obesity health risks, and obesity among Black African immigrants living in the US. Even though acculturation did not significantly predict increased obesity health risk symptoms, increased resilience significantly predicted decreased obesity health risk symptoms. In addition, resilience moderated between acculturation and obesity health risk symptoms. Higher levels of resilience were associated with fewer obesity health risk symptoms when the participant also had high acculturation levels. Additional results showed that neither acculturation nor resilience significantly predicted obesity, respectively. Furthermore, resilience did not moderate between acculturation and obesity.

Finally, one of the most significant contributions of this study was its examination of the constructs of acculturation, resilience, obesity health risks, and obesity outcomes among Black African immigrants using Gallo and Matthew's (2003) RCM theoretical framework, which has never been done before. Therefore, this study has contributed to the theoretical base of the RCM. There are many implications of this research in that it can be used to create programs to establish resilience building training for immigrant communities, and it can be used to create educational programs to reduce the number of health related risks which could then reduce reliance on governmental healthcare. Future studies could examine obesity and obesity health risks over time in relation to the constructs of acculturation and resilience, and also include the examination of other cultural factors, such as the individual's native country, that may be associated with obesity and health problems related to obesity.